Clinical Aspects of Sleep and Sleep Disturbance

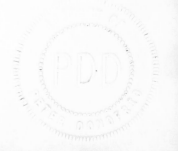

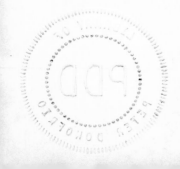

Clinical Aspects of Sleep and Sleep Disturbance

Edited by
Terrence L. Riley, M.D.

Director, Division of Neurology,
Quincy City Hospital,
Quincy, Massachusetts

With 5 Contributing Authors

BUTTERWORTH PUBLISHERS
Boston • London
Sydney • Wellington • Durban • Toronto

*Every effort has been made to ensure that the drug dosage sched-
ules within this text are accurate and conform to standards accepted
at time of publication. However, as treatment recommendations
vary in light of continuing research and clinical experience, the
reader is advised to verify drug dosage schedules herein with information found on product information sheets. This is especially
true in cases of new or infrequently used drugs.*

Library of Congress Cataloging in Publication Data
Main entry under title:

Clinical aspects of sleep and sleep disturbance.

  Includes index.
  1. Sleep disorders. 2. Sleep. I. Riley, Terrence L.
[DNLM: 1. Sleep—Physiology. 2. Sleep disorders. WM 188
C641]
RC547.C55 1984   616.8'49   84–3220
ISBN 0–409–95071–8

Butterworth Publishers
80 Montvale Avenue
Stoneham, MA 02180

10 9 8 7 6 5 4 3 2 1

Printed in the United States of America.

To James D. Dexter, who taught me the thrill of medical inquiry, and to William L. Brannon, Jr., who taught me how to be a neurologist.

CONTENTS

CONTRIBUTING AUTHORS

Richard Ferber, M.D.
Instructor in Medicine,
Harvard Medical School;
Director, Sleep Disorders Clinic,
Children's Hospital
Medical Center,
Boston, Massachusetts

Ramon Greenberg, M.D.
Visiting Professor
Harvard Medical School,
Brookline, Massachusetts

Peter J. Hauri, Ph.D.
Associate Professor of Psychiatry
(Clinical Psychology),
Dartmouth Medical School;
Director, Dartmouth-Hitchcock
Sleep Clinic,
Hanover, New Hampshire

George F. Howard III, M.D.
Acting Director,
EEG and Sleep Laboratories,
University Hospital,
Boston, Massachusetts

William C. Orr, Ph.D.
Director, Sleep Laboratory,
University of Oklahoma/
Presbyterian Hospital,
Oklahoma City, Oklahoma

PREFACE

The topic of sleep is one of those catchy subjects that has attracted a good deal of public attention lately, and for which sleep clinics and a burgeoning specialty of science is emerging. There are at least two major professional societies dedicated to the study of sleep and regulation of sleep centers. There is a certification board not only for sleep (polysomnography) technologists, but also for physicians and PhDs who run such centers and laboratories. The importance of sleep disturbances to the public is evident in the large market for medications, both in prescription and over-the-counter forms, that enable people to fall asleep or stay asleep.

Even with several current journals to review sleep research and recent books about sleep disturbances, most available literature is directed either toward lay magazines on the one hand or to sleep researchers on the other. Practicing clinicians have often been ignored. Indeed, the primary physician, psychiatrist, or neurologist not uncommonly has the feeling that sleep problems all need to be referred to one of the few certified sleep laboratories where a sleep specialist takes over. Undoubtedly, there are cases of sufficient complexity that only a person with special expertise and the leisure of time afforded by a referral center can deal with them appropriately. Such hoarding or sequestering of particular clinical complaints, however, only serves to make sleeping disorders a greater burden for the patient unnecessarily referred elsewhere. People may be discouraged from appropriate treatment. The concept that only the "ivory tower" can take care of difficult problems is outdated.

This book attempts to provide for the practicing clinician, whether in pediatrics, family practice, neurology, psychiatry, or other medical specialties, the information needed to take an intelligent history and deal with most problems of sleeping and waking encountered in office or hospital practice. We feel a discussion of the biological organization of sleep is necessary as a foundation for understanding pathophysiology and treatment. The peculiar sleeping and waking problems of childhood and adolescence are discussed in a separate chapter, but some effort has been made to integrate these with the particular problems facing people of all ages. The "primary" sleep disorders such as narcolepsy and nocturnal myoclonus are covered in a separate chapter from the consideration of sleep problems in medical and surgical practice. Insomnia rivals constipation and headache as the most common complaint in doctors' offices. It is discussed here together with the other "primary sleep disturbances," those disorders of the sleep-wake cycle not immediately attributable to other disease states. Although there is some discussion of hypnotics, we have not provided "guidelines" or prescriptions for how to select a particular agent for the individual patient. While this is tempting, it is necessary to individualize treatment. To avoid the hazards of addiction, respiratory embarrassment, and mental status changes from unwise use of hypnotics, we have instead chosen to outline the causes and approaches to insomnia and to provide principles by which an intelligent physician can solve the prescribing problem just as he or she would for infection, heart failure, or any other medical disease.

Above all, it is our goal to show that understanding the sleep-wake cycle and approaching the clinical challenge of sleeping and waking disturbances are not mystical enterprises. Rather, the same principles of history taking and assessing the patient's environment that would be important for a complaint of headache pertain also to the evaluation of sleep disturbances. We have sufficient technological wherewithal now that appropriate laboratory studies can help us more precisely characterize the causes of the patient's symptoms and help us to measure responses to therapy. But this does not replace history taking. Basic principles of medicine are appropriate here, as they are for the complaint of cough or stomach pain. It is our intention to provide the background and principles that will enable the physician to deal with these issues.

My thanks to Sara Crafts, Susan Norman, Julie A. Hayes, and Wesley Paul for their kind assistance in the preparation of this manuscript.

T.L.R.

Clinical Aspects of Sleep and Sleep Disturbance

CHAPTER 1

Historical Overview and Introduction
Terrence L. Riley

Apparently the earliest concept of sleep was a "retreat" of the spirit from the body, permitting communion with other spirits or possession by supernatural forces. In such an ethereal state, ideas, virtues, or evil motives could be instilled or the body could simply be nourished. Eventually, when the brain was recognized as the seat of consciousness, this mythological interpretation surrendered to the "deafferentation" theory. Simply stated, this hypothesis concludes that the brain cannot stay awake if it is disconnected from afferent sensory input. In 1809 Rolando removed the cerebrum from birds and noted that the creatures behaved as though asleep. Currently, this might be looked on as a naïve experiment, but the validity of the observation (if not the conclusion) is unquestioned. Purkinje, noting the results of Rolando and Flourens, concluded in 1845 that sleep was the resulting state when the brainstem and the localizing cerebral systems were lost anywhere along a path between brainstem and cortex. A constant flow of afferent impulses from the body was considered necessary for maintaining wakefulness. So severing of such incoming messages defaulted the waking state and left the organism asleep. In this model, sleep would be interpreted as a kind of unresponsiveness, a resting state of the whole body resulting from "turning off" wakefulness (O'Leary and Goldring, 1976).

Even before the advent of modern physiological methods, however, there were observations that showed that sleep had to be more than an extreme form of inactivity. Griesinger (1868) noted that in sleeping humans and mammals, rapid eye movements under the closed lids coincided with twitching movements of the body. He concluded that this form of activity during sleep was somehow connected to dreams. Certainly, since antiquity, speech during dreams and increased autonomic activity during sleep were subjects of much speculation and rich literature.

Simply by observing people in sleep, before electroencephalographic (EEG) manifestations of sleep were clarified, MacWilliam (1920) demonstrated that changes in blood pressure, pulse, respiration, and other autonomic manifestations such as penile erections occurred episodically and predictably during the night.

1

Studies of diseases provided early examples of altered sleep-wake cycles and suggested some of the physiological mechanisms involved in integrating sleep and wakefulness. During the pandemic viral encephalitis in 1918 to 1920, von Economo predicted that lesions in the hypothalamus would account for disturbance of wakefulness and sleep; these were later identified by Nauta anatomically (Bremer, 1974, 1980; von Economo, 1929). Von Economo described two neuropathological syndromes affecting wakefulness, one resulting in excessive somnolence and the other in sleeplessness, or profound insomnia. He showed that structural lesions in the midbrain tegmentum and posterior hypothalamus seemed to result in the drowsy or somnolent state, whereas lesions of the basal forebrain and striatum led to insomnia (1929).

In 1929 Hans Berger demonstrated spontaneous oscillations of brain electrical potentials, revolutionizing the field of neurological diagnosis and providing the greatest tool to study states of brain activity. Modern understanding and experimental approaches to sleep might truly be said to begin with this work. Shortly after Berger demonstrated the alpha rhythm, EEG correlations with states of arousal were demonstrated. Hess (1929) demonstrated that electrical activation in certain brain centers, usually the brainstem, could cause an animal to sleep, but only with certain stimulation at a few specific frequencies.

Despite the growing physiological evidence that sleep was in fact dependent upon intrinsic regulating mechanisms, one of the next key observations paradoxically resurrected the older deafferentation theory. When Bremer sectioned the brainstem at midbrain level, below the oculomotor nucleus, or between the superior and inferior colliculi (cerveau isolé), he caused a state of permanent sleep, with high-voltage slow waves in the electrocorticogram, divergence of the eyes, and pupillary constriction. This seemed to show that sleep indeed was a result of isolation or deafferentation of the cerebrum: isolate cerebrum from brainstem and permanent sleep results.

Things became a good deal more complicated when sections between the medulla and cervical spine or transection of the brainstem at the base of the skull (encéphale isolé) produced permanent wakefulness, an animal who could not sleep (Battini, Magni, Paletini, et al, 1959; Battini, Moruzzi, Paletini, et al, 1958). Bremer, Jouvet, and others realized that the problem was more complicated than an on-off toggle switch. A caudal brainstem mechanism seemed responsible for induction of sleep, while wakefulness depended in part on an activating system between the upper midbrain and the cerebral hemispheres.

The landmark studies of Moruzzi and Magoun (1949) demonstrated the importance of the reticular activating system, with projection of ascending reticular neurons to cerebral hemispheres. These authors demonstrated that rapid, repetitive stimuli of reticular core neurons in the midbrain would result in activation of cortical neurons. Destruction of the reticular core led to an unresponsive cortex—a somnolent animal—and rendered the cortical neurons unresponsive to activation when reticular core neurons were subsequently stimulated by a frequency previously capable of inducing cortical excitability. From this, Moruzzi (1964) developed the critical recognition that in the alert animal, the cerebral cortex is maintained in a state of activation by a steady afferent volley along spinal reticulocerebral-activating systems, which exert a facilitating influence on the cerebrum necessary to maintain wakefulness. Loss of this facilitation allows vigilance to drop below a certain critical level and permits the organism to "fall asleep." This was a more complicated reason than before, but still a deafferentation schema.

These initial observations of the function of the reticular activating system are still pertinent to our current understanding of sleep mechanisms and constitute all that many practicing physicians know about regulating wakefulness or sleep (Kales, Kales, Bixler, et al, 1980).

The deafferentation hypothesis was dealt a blow only eight years after Berger described the EEG when Loomis, Harvey, and Hobart (1937) described distinguishable EEG patterns during sleep that were not seen during wakefulness. Because of differences in patterns, stages were labeled A, B, C, D, and E, depending upon persistence or voltage of alpha rhythms (stage A), suppression of voltage and elimination of alpha rhythm (stage B), occurrence of rhythmical central spindle waves (stage C), and diffuse high-voltage slow waves (stage E). An intermediate stage characterized by the persistence of central spindle waves with interspersed high-voltage slow waves was called stage D. Since the brain waves were characterized by apparently organized alterations of physiological markers during sleep, it became more and more apparent that sleep was not simply a passive state of deafferentation. When Aserinsky and Kleitman in 1953 demonstrated that episodic rapid eye movements occurred with dreaming and the recall of dreams (noted 90 years earlier by Griesinger), it was finally apparent that sleep as an integrated physiological event was much more complicated than simply turning off the brain. By the 1950s electrophysiological techniques were adequate for simultaneously recording brain waves, body movement, and many other physiological events. This soon led to a large body of information about physiological concomitants of sleep. In the ensuing 25 years, much has been learned about several primary stages of sleep, although most of what has been reported still remains scattered descriptions of behavioral and physiological phenomena and epiphenomena, often without explanations or understanding of the biological basis of these phenomena.

THE PURPOSE OF SLEEP

Remarkably, despite the complicated studies of the physiology and behaviors observed in sleep, the purpose of sleep for the organism or the psyche remains enigmatic. While it appears that rapid eye movement (REM) sleep is necessary to maintain a certain integrity of neuronal excitability, and while slow wave sleep seems to have an important influence on the musculoskeletal system, it is not even clear what the various long-recognized stages accomplish. Indeed, why do we even need different stages? While there remains considerable uncertainty about the respective biological functions of the several stages of sleep, it appears that slow wave sleep accomplishes some form of physical musculoskeletal restorative function and that REM sleep in some manner provides a form of recovery of higher mental function or neuronal stability (see Chapter 3 under "Biological Stages of Sleep"). The overall function or value of sleep remains less clear. The only universally agreed-upon result of sleep deprivation is feeling sleepy. In other words, the most certain reason for sleep is to avoid being sleepy. How painfully circuitous.

The two most attractive explanations for the necessity of sleep can be called a *restorative theory* and an *ethological/conservation theory*. They probably are perfectly compatible and need not be seen as either mutually exclusive or as one theory being a better explanation than the other.

Most consistent with our intuitive feelings about sleep are the arguments for the restorative theory. Oswald (1980) concedes that sleep may have a protective value, as a conservation theory suggests, but he argues that it has most significantly an indispensible role in tissue restoration. During sleeping hours there is a shift in the balance between protein synthesis and degradation toward more synthetic functions. Among mammals, brain protein synthesis, nucleic acid synthesis throughout the body, and brain adenosine triphosphate all achieve higher levels during sleep or in the customary sleeping periods (Adams, 1980). In humans, more amino acids are liberated in the hours 8 through 11 PM than during the sleeping hours of 2 to 5 AM even during total dietary starvation. Sleep deprivation leads to higher excretion of the catecholamines that have catabolic functions, and also to negative nitrogen balance, implying that without sleep, there is a loss of protein or a shift back to catabolism. Adams and Oswald (1977) and Adams (1980) summarize some of the most important arguments for the restorative thesis: there are more mitoses in actively dividing cell lines during sleep, including kidney, intestine, and skin; species metabolic rates correlate with sleep (animals with higher rates of oxidative metabolism sleep longer than those with lower oxidative rates); the anabolic hormones (growth hormone, corticosteroids, and gonadotropin) predominate during sleeping hours, but catabolic hormones (such as catecholamines) predominate during waking hours.

In the restorative argument it is generally conceded that slow wave sleep is "worth more" in the physical restorative process. After periods of total deprivation, the first recovery sleep preferentially has a rebound of slow wave sleep. Physical exercise may cause measurable subsequent awareness of sleepiness (Lubin, Hord, Tracy, et al, 1976) and preferentially increases slow wave sleep when sleep is allowed (Griffin and Trinder, 1978).

The same amount of physical exercise among nonathletic subjects also leads to associated elevations of growth hormone release (Adamson, Hunter, Ogundremi, et al, 1974). Dieting or fasting also increases the total amount of slow wave sleep (Karacan, Rosenbloom, Londono, et al, 1973), which may be considered a compensatory attempt to restore or preserve protein in the starving animal, if in fact slow wave sleep has a restorative function.

Moruzzi (1966) and others have argued that the neuronal or psychic restorative processes of REM sleep may provide a subtler form of restoration for psychological well-being. In the sense of sorting memories that should be recalled or arranging cortical priorities to experiences of the preceding waking interval, then the psychological restorative processes may reside particularly in REM or paradoxical sleep in animals.

An ethological or conservation theory has also been proposed to explain the need for sleep. It is apparent that species survival or prosperity may depend in animals as complicated as the human or as simple as the amoeba upon synchronizing food-seeking behaviors and the guidance systems of the organism with the heat and light cycles of the planet and with the levels of vulnerability or availability of prey or other members of the species.

Since we live on a planet with daily cycles of changing degrees of temperature and light, efficient survival or maximal well-being may depend on synchronizing our activity with these cycles. For many animals, feeding is most efficient in daylight, and a period of relative inactivity when feeding is inefficient should conserve energy stores. Although sleep is an energy-consuming mechanism in the brain, overall body metabolism and energy use are clearly diminished during sleep in mammals and birds (Allison and Van Twyer, 1970). It would be an oversimplification to look at sleep behavior simply as energy-consuming, however. For animals who depend on the daylight for guidance, such as horses and humans, to walk about in the dark may predispose to injury or expose the organism to predators. Sleep forces a protective inactivity.

Our functions vary with the seasons in most climates of earth, also. Since the length of daylight dictates temperature and, for the most part, food supplies, it is efficient for most large land animals to have dormant periods when longer nights and colder weather predominate. It is during such seasons that both vegetable and animal foodstuffs are less plentiful, and energy conservation while sleeping tucked away in a cave or hovel is advantageous to survival. Sleeping favors survival not only by encouraging use of the nest to avoid hypothermia. When depletion of foliage diminishes hiding spaces or camouflage, staying asleep lowers exposure to predators.

The so-called dream state generator (Hobson and McCarley, 1977; Hobson, McCarley, and Wyzinski, 1975) may be invoked to explain either the ethological/conservation model or the restorative model. In many regards the restorative process as argued by Oswald and others could actually be best accomplished in an energy-conserving model of the ethological theory. Other derivative explanations for the functions of sleep have been suggested, including a protective theory, which basically argues that neuronal protection may be afforded by periodic inactivity; and an instinctive theory proposing that a species-specific innate pattern of behavior similar to nest building, which is inborn in many species, dictates a particular sleeping pattern.

All of these explanations of the purposes or functions of sleep have some flaws. If all birds and mammals not only sleep, but have REM/non-REM cycles, why should those different species have the same instincts for different sleep stages? As regards the ethological/conservation theory, not all birds and mammals live in fluctuating light and dark environments. For example, some dwell in dark environments, some only in tropical settings, and others in subterranean environments in which significant changes in temperature or light do not occur. Sleep would seem to have, for example, little benefit for a mole, yet he sleeps. So, while the basic need or purpose of sleep remains a mystery, it is clear that there are several benefits to the organism from sleeping, and the various functions are not always closely intertwined. Rechtschaffen and associates (1983) deprived 8 rats of sleep for 5 to 33 days. They all developed ataxia, yellow fever, and swelling of paws. Three died after 5, 13, and 33 days, and four others were sacrificed when EEG voltage dropped and they appeared moribund. No single fatal pathological lesion was found grossly or microscopically at necropsy. Pulmonary fluid, internal hemorrhage, and testicular edema were seen. Similar evidence of the impact of sleep deprivation is not yet confirmed in humans or other species. A form of restoration must at least be present in humans, and even a kind of protective benefit, because of the recognized need for sleep and the age-old applicability in all languages of the very word *sleepiness*.

REFERENCES

Adams K. Sleep as a restorative process and theory to explain why. Prog Brain Res 1980;53:289–325.

Adams K, Oswald I. Sleep is for tissue restoration. J Coll Physicians 1977;11:376–88.

Adamson L, Hunter WM, Ogundremi O, Oswald I, Percy-Robb I. Growth hormone increase during sleep after daytime exercise. J Endocrinol 1974;62:473–78.

Allison T, Van Twyer H. The evolution of sleep. Natural Hist 1970;79:56–65.

Aserinsky E, Kleitman N. Regularly occurring periods of eye motility and concomitant phenomena during sleep. Science 1953;118:273–74.

Battini C, Magni F, Paletini M, Rossi GF, Zanchetti M. Neuronal mechanisms underlying EEG and behavioral activation in the midpontine pretrigeminal cat. Arch Ital Biol 1959;13–25.

Battini C, Moruzzi G, Paletini M, Rossi GF, Zanchetti A. Persistent patterns of wakefulness in the pretrigeminal midpontine preparation. Science 1958;128:30–32.

Berger H. Über das Elektroenkephalogramm des Menschen. Arch Psychiatr Nervenkr 1929;87:527.

Bremer F. Historical development in ideas on sleep. In: Petre-Quadens O, Schlag JD, eds. Basic sleep mechanisms. New York: Academic Press, 1974:3–11.

Bremer F. Biology of sleep. Experientia 1980;36:1–5.

Griesinger W. Berliner medizinisch-psychologische Gesellschaft. Arch Psychiatr Nervenkr 1868;1:200–4.

Griffin SJ, Trinder J. Physical fitness, exercise, and human sleep. Soc Psychophysiol Res 1978;15(5):447–50.

Hess WR. Hirn Reizversuche über Mechanismus des Schlafes. Arch Psychiatr Nervenkr 1929;86:287–92.

Hobson J, McCarley R. The brain as a dream state generator: an activation-synthesis hypothesis of the dream process. Am J Psychiatry 1977;134:1335–48.

Hobson JA, McCarley RW, Wyzinski P. Sleep cycle oscillation: reciprocal discharge by two brainstem neuronal groups. Science 1975;189:55–58.

Kales JD, Kales A, Bixler EO, Soldatos CR. Sleep disorders: what the primary care physician needs to know. Postgrad Med 1980;67(3):213–17.

Karacan I, Rosenbloom I, Londono J, Salis, Thornby J, Williams R. The effect of acute fasting on sleep and the sleep growth hormone response. Psychosomatics 1973;14:33–37.

Loomis AL, Harvey EN, Hobart GA. Cerebral states during sleep, as studied by human brain potentials. J Exp Physiol 1937;21:127–44.

Lubin A, Hord D, Tracy M, Johnson L. Effects of exercise, bedrest, and napping on performance decrement during 40 hours. Psychophysiology 1976;13:334–39.

MacWilliam JA. Some applications of physiology to medicine. III. Blood pressure and heart action in sleep and dreams. Br Med J 1920;II:1196–1200.

Moruzzi G. The historical development of the deafferentation hypothesis of sleep. Proc Am Philos Soc 1964;108:19–28.

Moruzzi G. The functional significance of sleep with particular regard to the brain mechanisms underlying consciousness. In: Eccles, J, ed. Brain and conscious experience. New York: Springer, 1966.

Moruzzi G, Magoun H. Brainstem reticular formation and activation of the EEG. Electroencephalogr Clin Neurophysiol 1949;1:455–73.

O'Leary J, Goldring S. Science and epilepsy. New York: Raven Press, 1976;164–65.

Oswald I. Sleep, the great restorer. New Sci 1970;46:170–72.

Oswald I. Sleep as a restorative process: human clues. Prog Brain Res 1980;53:279–88.

Purkinje D. Wachen Schlaf Traum und verwandte zustande. In: H.P. von Wagner, ed. Handworterbuch der Physiologie. Vol. 2 Braunschweig, Vieweg & Sohn, 1846:412–80.

Rechtschaffen A, Gilliland MA, Bergmann BM, Winter JB. Physiological correlates of prolonged sleep deprivation in rats. Science 1983;221:182–84.

von Economo C. Schlaftheorie. Ergeb Physiol 1929;28:312–39.

PART I

Normal Sleep

CHAPTER 2

Biological Organization
of Sleep
Terrence L. Riley

This chapter concerns the anatomical and physiological factors that govern sleep; Chapter 3 considers behavioral aspects of sleep. An attempt to describe physiological or chemical mechanisms as though separate from behaviors or functions runs the risk of simply cataloging a series of observations and missing the opportunity to bridge the theories. Certainly, behavior is not only the result of biophysical action on substrates, and the reverse is also true: biochemical functions often *depend* upon environmental cues or behavioral motivations. There is some redundancy in these two chapters, but our aim is to provide several perspectives on the functions that occur during sleep and on how certain life and body functions are affected by different phases of the sleep-wake cycle. The attempt is not to fragment these concepts or to imply that one perspective can truly be seen independently from the other. Some readers, however, will not be as interested in neuroanatomy or biochemistry. Also, the integration of different behaviors or various anatomical systems may be lost in excessive detail if all paragraphs try to cover all aspects. Finally, the complete synthesis or understanding of some whole systems is not yet at hand. It is more accurate sometimes to report observations than to posit premature theories.

ANATOMICAL FACTORS

Cajal (1952) described several important considerations in terms of brainstem structure that have proved critical in the understanding of sleep regulation. First, the giant cells in the paramedian reticular formation of the midbrain and superior pons, also called gigantocellular neurons and collectively called field tegmentogigantocellularis (FTG), have projections to many areas, especially along paramidline pathways and reticular formation structures. Second, the raphe neurons running midline along the entire brainstem, but heaviest in the medulla, are connected in a manner that allows effective regulation of other paramedian elements that also project throughout the brain. Finally, Cajal suggested that the input to the central reticular core might be from small stellate cells located more lateral in the brainstem. Such an input channel recognized diffusely throughout the brainstem and spinal cord and with spread into superior regions of the brain might be influential not only to modulate a core oscillator to stimulus cues, but perhaps to abort the firing of a trigger oscillator system. Cajal's earlier studies were amplified by the work of others (Brodal, 1957; Scheibel and Scheibel, 1967) showing that both spinal cord and thalamus received widespread projects from the FTG neurons. These neurons synapse widely in cerebral cortex in frontal, parietal, and occipital areas, directly on oculomotor nucleus in midbrain, and on both lower motoneurons and presumed inhibitory interneurons in ventral horn of spinal cord. Although apparently few in number, the FTG neurons by virtue of size probably have enormous synaptic ramifications, each likely projecting to 9 million postsynaptic membranes. In other words, if there were 3,000 cells in the cat FTG, this might account for several billion synapses along both ascending and descending pathways.

Classic sensory pathways were once thought to be responsible for maintaining wakefulness; sleep, as a kind of deafferentation of the cortex, was the state resulting from the interruption or collapse of sensory stimulation to the cortex. Moruzzi and Magoun (1949) showed that the extralemniscal reticular formation was able to elicit arousal from sleep, accompanied by desynchronization of the electroencephalogram (EEG) (rapid but varying frequencies of low amplitude in the EEG). Such stimulation studies enhanced Bremer's earlier observations (see Chapter 1) that wakefulness was sacrificed by isolating the forebrain from brainstem with an intracollicular section and that transection of the stem below the locus ceruleus, at pontomedullary level resulted in a state of hyperalertness, or insomnia. Battini, Magni, Paletini, et al (1959) noted that complete pontine transection not only caused excessive alertness, but produced repetitive, phasic ocular movements suggestive of rapid eye movement (REM) sleep.

Large lesions of the pontine reticular formation eliminate desynchronized or paradoxical sleep (Jouvet, 1962) and yet transactions above the pons or complete ablation of the forebrain do not affect the periodicity of paradoxical sleep or the duration of muscular or ocular manifestations of paradoxical sleep in animals. The conclusions from such studies are that the trigger, the generator, and the timing mechanism for paradoxical sleep phases must reside within the area of ablation, the pons. Small lesions of the anterior or dorsal pons that ablate the locus ceruleus usually eliminate the atonia characteristic of paradoxical sleep in cats, but not other features of this state (Jouvet and Delorme, 1965; Hobson and McCarley, 1975; McCarley, 1981). With more precise dissection, ablation, or stimulation of the locus ceruleus, Jouvet (1967a&b) concluded that the caudal two-thirds of the locus ceruleus was responsible for inhibition of muscle tone during paradoxical (REM) sleep, and the medial or anterior one-third was more responsible for aspects such as cortical activation (desynchronization) on EEG and phasic events such as rapid eye movements and integrated discharges in pons, geniculate ganglia, and cortex (pontine-geniculate-occipital spikes).

Certainly the functions of sleep are not limited to the brainstem. As Freud and most other observers have recognized since nearly a century ago, the cerebral hemispheres and especially the cortex clearly undergo significant transformations during sleep. Since sensory imagery and emotions are generally conceded either to reside in or at least incorporate cortical functions, and since sensory imagery and emotions account for the most striking features of dreams, it is clear that the cortex must be actively involved in sleep regulation, at least in dreaming. Early investigations into the brain centers responsible for the jerking body movements and movements of animals' whiskers, paws, and eyes during paradoxical sleep found that immediately before such movements, electrographical discharges, or spikes, could be recorded sequentially from pons, lateral geniculate ganglion, and occipital cortex. These were termed pontine-geniculate-occipital (PGO) spikes (Jouvet, 1962, 1969; Jeannerod, Mouret, and Jouvet, 1965; Roffwarg, Dement, and Muzio, 1962). Jouvet noted that the PGO spikes occurred in rabbits at a fairly constant rate during paradoxical sleep, about 60 times per minute, and also continued throughout a 24-hour period averaging 14,000 spikes per day (range, 11,000 to 17,000). Earliest conclusions that the pontine trigger of PGO spikes emanated from FTG have given way to speculation that the spikes could derive from discharges in the anteromedial one-third of the locus ceruleus. It may be that the spikes simultaneously produce eye movements, cortical activation, and vestibular stimulation. Viewing the locus ceruleus/FTG axis as a dream state generator, the Hobson-McCarley model suggests that dreams are the "explanation" humans give to the level of brain activation resulting from REM sleep, rather than a psychodynamic experience.

In one of the earliest reports of evoked potentials during sleep, Shagass and Trusty (1967) showed that a continuous tendency of briefer latencies to both somatosensory and visual evoked potentials occurred only when REM sleep occurred in temporal sequences between stages I and II. Cerebral evoked responses in lower mammals have had generally higher voltages and shorter latencies in paradoxical sleep than slow wave sleep. This is further evidence of a state of cortical excitation or activation during REM or paradoxical sleep.

Initiation of Sleep: Hypothalamic Factors

The duration of effect of currently recognized neurotransmitters in brainstem sleep centers is too brief to account for ultradian sleep-wake cycles. Phase adjustments and responsiveness to environmental or dietary change must require longer or slower effects.

As early as 1929, Fulton and Ingraham noted that lesions in the prechiasmatic regions of the hypothalamus were able to induce not only emotional disturbances and hyperexcitability, but marked disturbances in sleep-wake cycles and in fact, chronic insomnia. Nauta (1946) showed that specific lesions in anterior hypothalamus destroyed sleep regulation in rats and resulted often in sleepless animals.

Stimulation of the preoptic forebrain regions in cats and monkeys, near the region of suprachiasmatic or supraoptic nuclei, has been shown not only to cause cortical EEG synchronization (slow waves), but clear behavioral inhibition and a state resembling slow wave sleep (Clemente, 1969; Clemente, Sterman, and Wyrwicka, 1963). Although the giant cells of the pontine tegmentum with the greatest increase in discharge rates during REM sleep vary firing rate continuously (Hobson, McCarley, Freedman, and Pivik, 1974; Hobson, McCarley, and Freedman, 1974), there are particularly striking changes in firing rates just before the EEG becomes desynchronized during REM, just before clusters of rapid eye movements, and before shifts in body tone or posture. Koella (1967) argues that, in addition to the centers responsible for the integration and organization of sleep sequences, there may be a function of midline thalamic nuclei that contributes to sleep induction, but such a thalamic role remains speculative. The midline thalamic complexes may be considered deactivating systems that must be responsible for dampening the reticular gating system in order that the sleep-inducing systems may emerge, as though there were two coordinated antagonistic systems.

Moore and Eichler (1976) found that lesions of the suprachiasmatic nucleus in the anterior hypothalamus abolished a wide array of circadian rhythms, including the sleep-wake cycle. Using deoxyglucose labeled with carbon 14, it has recently been found that the suprachiasmatic nucleus is much more active metabolically in animals living in a light/dark circadian environment than in those kept constantly in darkness (Schwartz and Gainer, 1981). The suprachiasmatic nucleus regulates not only diurnal feeding patterns but onset of sleep. The capability of adapting to shifts in light and dark sequences in the circadian cycle also is a function of the suprachiasmatic nucleus. The suprachiasmatic nucleus does receive direct synaptic input from optic tract fibers, apparently independent of the geniculocalcarine pathway. This pathway conveys light/dark information directly from the retina to the suprachiasmatic nucleus (Moore, 1979) by way of monosynaptic connections (the retinohypothalamic tract) (Rusak and Zucker, 1979; Lydic, Schoene, Czeisler, et al, 1980).

In humans there is not as distinct a structure as the suprachiasmatic nucleus in smaller mammals, but there is a small, loosely packed cluster of neurons in the hypothalamus above the optic chiasm that appears comparable to the suprachiasmatic nucleus in primates. The cluster in humans is small, with diffuse boundaries, so there remains some controversy as to the role of this nucleus for regulation of circadian rhythms in man (Lydic et al, 1980). Another reason for controversy about the suprachiasmatic nucleus in humans is that at least 12 different terms have been used to identify the cluster of neurons since its first discovery in 1888, confounding attempts to follow investigations reported in the literature over time. Significant phylogenetic differences in the shape of the optic recess overlying the chiasm make direct anatomical comparisons between humans and other mammals difficult. Finally, a structure-function relationship has only recently been recognized for the suprachiasmatic nucleus even for lower mammals, so that such a function could not have been recognized earlier in humans.

The specific neuronal anastomoses or neurotransmitters used by a hypothalamic mechanism to regulate sleep phases are as yet unclear. Peptide transmitters have been identified as releasing hormones from many hypothalamic nuclei in pituitary and other endocrine functions, and have recently been implicated in sleep onset. Hypothalamic functions may have escaped detection for so many years because their messengers, the neuropeptides, act at widely distributed sites rather than at definable synaptic sites. Such wide-ranging influences from the hypothalamus may link environmental, emotional, or cortical needs to brainstem mechanisms for the regulation of sleep.

INTERACTING REGULATORS

Hobson, McCarley, and Freedman (1974) and Hobson et al (1974) showed that neurons in the FTG initiate a gradual increase in discharge rate five minutes before the onset of desynchronized (REM) sleep, and bursts of such discharges from FTG neurons were followed by rapid eye movements within 250 msec. These findings led to the conclusion that FTG neurons were a critical part of the pacing or regulating system for desynchronized sleep. Because many locus ceruleus (LC) neurons had high concentrations of norepinephrine and other catecholamines, the authors explored the possible interaction or reciprocal relationship between LC cells and those of the phasic regular discharging rates from FTG neurons.

By recording extracellular action potentials from individual nerve cells in cats, they found that the discharge density of certain cells in the LC had a reciprocal relationship with those in the FTG, but there were two kinds of cells in the LC with differential effects on the FTG. A minority of cells shared with other pontine brainstem neurons a weakly increased rate of discharge during desynchronized (REM) sleep. A remarkably different group, by far the majority in the LC of cats, had a strongly negative correlation. The trend of accelerating or decelerating discharge rate of majority population of LC cells was reciprocal, opposite, to the trend of acceleration and deceleration in the FTG cells: when the LC neuronal discharge rate diminished, the FTG neuronal discharge rate and amplitude were augmented, as though uninhibited or released (Figure 2.1).

Hobson and co-workers concluded that reciprocal interaction between the interconnected cell populations was in large measure responsible for the

ANATOMY OF SLEEP REGULATION

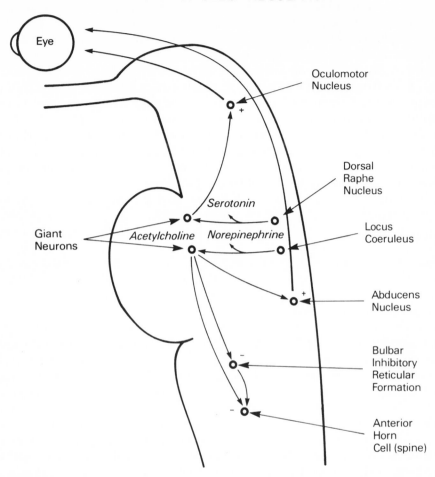

Figure 2.1.   Although the brain as a whole enters a unique state of activity during sleep, the reciprocal activities of the field gigantocellularis (giant neurons) in pons and midbrain, the midline raphe nuclei, and the locus ceruleus coordinate several elaborate pacemaker functions.

cyclical interaction of behavioral states. The primarily norepinephrine-containing neurons that are inhibitory to FTG neurons impair or terminate firing bursts from the FTG neurons, which pace or initiate REM epochs. Midline or dorsal raphe nuclei also seem to have negative input to the FTG. Both serotonin- and norepinephrine-containing neurons impinge upon FTG neurons, and when iontophoretically applied to FTG neurons, both serotonin and norepinephrine inhibit firing of FTG neurons. At sleep onset, as LC activity begins to wane, FTG neurons begin to fire progressively more rapidly and intensively. Having reached a certain degree of discharge or activity, in part enhanced by positive feedback reinforcement, FTG neurons escape LC inhibition and trigger the behavioral manifestations of desynchronized or paradoxical sleep (REM). Progressively increased discharging rates from the FTG then trigger further activation of LC, which eventually provides inhibitory feedback on FTG and terminates desynchronized sleep (Hobson, McCarley, and Wyzinsky, 1975).

Following the demonstration that cell groups in the LC and FTG fulfill reciprocal oscillatory inhibition/excitation coupling, McCarley and Hobson explored a mathematical interaction between the two groups of cells. If X(T) is considered the level of discharge activity in FTG neurons; Y(T) the level of discharge activity in LC cells; and A, B, C, and D respectively represent positive constants representing the strength of connections between the cells, then the terms might be related by the following equation:

$$DX/DT = AX - BXY,$$
$$DY/DT = -CY + DXY.$$

This system of equations was originally proposed as a model for prey and predator interaction by Lotka and Volterra (Yamazaki, Ishikawa, Nakamura et al, 1979). It is suggested that the FTG excitatory neurons would be comparable to the susceptible prey population (X) and the inhibitory LC neurons comparable to the predators (Y) (McCarley and Hobson, 1975) in that activity or inactivity of one population would predictably and necessarily be accompanied by specific changes in activity of the other population.

In a subsequent review, Hobson, McCarley, and Wyzinski (1975) found that during the sleep cycle in cats, neurons localized to the posterolateral pole of the LC and the nucleus subceruleus undergo changes in discharge rate that are opposite the changes of the FTG neurons. The inverse rate ratios and activity curves of these two interconnected populations are compatible with reciprocal interaction as a physiological basis of sleep cycle oscillations. They constructed a model for the control of the desynchronized phase of sleep based on the reciprocal interaction between cells in the FTG and those of the posterolateral LC and the subceruleus. This physiological model reiterates the equation discussed above based on the Lotka-Volterra equations (Yamazaki et al, 1979).

It is important to remember that both monosynaptic and polysynaptic spinal reflexes are affected by fluctuations in the sleep-wake cycle (Pompeiano, 1967) and that in some ways they are more important for behavior than the ascending pathways from the brainstem to the cerebral cortex (Jouvet, 1962; Hobson and McCarley, 1977). For behavior or survival of the organisms, alterations in posture and body tone may be more critical than the state of cerebral activation.

In summary, the anatomical substrates of the regulation of sleep seem to be set in action by an ultradian or overall survival cycle likely to be regulated by suprachiasmatic nucleus. A priming or initiating center of sleep apparently resides in the midline raphe, particularly dorsal nuclei, of the medulla, with rostrally projecting "priming" input to the large neurons in the paramedian FTG. Once excited, FTG neurons crescendo in rate and intensity of discharge with excitatory synapses to cerebral cortical, oculomotor nucleus, and lateral geniculate nucleus and inhibitory synapses to spinal motor neuron and LC neurons. The LC in two poles seems to have in its posterolateral component a basic inhibitory population of neurons capable of suppressing FTG neurons until their crescendo firing rate escapes from the inhibition of LC neurons. As the discharge rate of a REM period reaches peak, selective neurons of LC inhibit the firing rate of FTG neurons, and either the raphe neurons increase in their function or the animal awakens (Hobson and McCarley, 1977).

NEUROTRANSMITTER FUNCTIONS IN
SLEEP-WAKE REGULATION

In the past 24 years the role of specific neurotransmitters and, more intriguingly, specific receptors on postsynaptic membranes have revolutionized our understanding of the nervous system. No longer can one look at the so-called dry circuits of any neurological function without considering the specific neurotransmitters that operate within that system. The subtle complexity of interactions of the transmitters and receptors enable adjacent sensitive neuronal systems to maintain high degrees of discrimination and specificity while functioning within microns of one another. It is not enough to identify various loci within the brainstem or hypothalamus, which, if ablated, interrupt the functions of sleep or any other behavior; nor is it sufficient to show that stimulation of these loci induces behavior. Many of the relevant neurotransmitters have been identified, and it is now possible to address with increasing accuracy the specific biochemical agents associated with any biological functions.

It is more or less possible to deal with the transmitters or modulators involved in wakefulness and sleep as though they were disembodied from the neurological anatomical structures responsible. To view the chemical structures without the context of their anatomical substrates would be imprecise and give a misleading impression of brain function. The neurotransmitters are not dissolved in an amorphous "soup" but are usually packaged, released, and active at discrete sites. Since one transmitter may accomplish different effects at different sites or in different amounts, it is important to remember that functional anatomy and neurochemistry really go hand in hand.

One must also consider neuromediators or regulator systems that have slower response curves and generally wider distribution, often by diffusion. Neurotransmitters may induce arousal or suppression by immediate stimulation from synaptic depolarization or hyperpolarization, and yet the modulators do not operate directly on receptors sites at a single site but render widespread sites more or less vulnerable to the specific transmitters that reach them.

Biogenic Amines

Serotonin

Elucidation of the function of serotonin (5-hydroxytryptamine, 5HT) in sleep has depended on classic methods of studying neurotransmitters: lesions of the nuclei containing the compound and pharmacological impairment of the primary compound metabolism. The primary cells that synthesize serotonin are for the most part localized in the midline or median raphe nuclei of the brainstem, all the way to the more rostral portions of the midbrain. With coagulation of the system, the animal is rendered unable to sleep, and a rather permanent state of behavioral wakefulness can be recorded both by EEG and by observation. Although there is rough correlation with the degree of insomnia and the amount of damage to the raphe lesion or loss of serotonin rostral to the lesion (Monnier and Gaillard, 1980), partial recovery may occur with time. In fact there are subsections of the raphe nuclei that have differential effects on sleep in general. Destruction of their anterior portion induces permanent wakefulness, but paradoxical sleep still appears during 5 to 10 percent of a 24-hour period without being preceded by slow wave sleep. By contrast, destruction of the posterior raphe nuclei does not eliminate non-REM (NREM) sleep but only reduces it to about 40 percent less than control; paradoxical sleep is completely abolished. The conclusion is that there is specialization within the raphe nuclei of the brainstem, with the anterior portion responsible for non-REM sleep and the posterior portion involved with a priming mechanism of paradoxical sleep.

Parachlorophenylalanine (PCPA) blocks tryptophan hydroxylase, the enzyme responsible for the primary rate-limiting step in the synthesis of serotonin. Although the administration of PCPA in man seems not to have significant effect, at least in cats and lower mammals it produces insomnia roughly paralleled by the degree of suppression of serotonin synthesis. In these conditions, large doses of 5-hydroxytryptophan, the precursor of serotonin, can overcome the block, and the animal can sleep. Concurrently, an effective block of serotonin by PCPA not only induces insomnia but blocks PGO spikes, the physiological signs of phasic components of REM sleep. Although serotonin usually restricts PGO spikes only to paradoxical sleep, PCPA may block the effects of serotonin on PGO spikes so that they intrude into NREM sleep and even wakefulness in animals.

Thus both ablation studies and pharmacological studies show that serotonin mechanisms may be responsible for maintaining NREM sleep and also play an important role in priming or regulating paradoxical sleep.

Catecholamines: Norepinephrine and Dopamine

Dopamine-containing cells in the locus ceruleus are responsible for the blue-black pigment for which the nucleus is named. It is recognized that in lesions of the LC resulting from either vascular interruption or degenerative processes that deplete the pigment-containing cells, there is disruption of the normal sleep sequence. Although the LC in mammals is only 3 to 5 mm in diameter, there are at least two major functional subsections, both primarily catecholaminergic. The anterior portion of the nucleus predominates in tonic cortical activation for wakefulness. When the dorsoanterior portion of the LC is ablated or isolated from neural connections, the resulting lesion produces hypersomnia, increasing both NREM sleep and paradoxical sleep in animals. With lesions of the dopamine-containing cells, which are primarily posteroventral, however, the animal has a generally motionless state, or akinesia, with normally alternating slow wave and waking EEG. Whether this represents a motor deficit analogous to a kind of parkinsonism, with depletion of dopamine from the cells responsible for motor movement, or a dopamine-dependent basis for maintaining wakefulness is not certain. Pharmacological blockade or stimulation of receptors for dopamine, however, influences central activation both in wakefulness and in paradoxical sleep. At any rate, there is clearly a correlation between brain catecholamines and paradoxical sleep. In fact, paradoxical sleep mechanisms require at least some degree of intact transmission between catecholamine synapses. When synthesis of norepinephrine is inhibited in cats by blocking tyrosine hydroxylase, the animals are immediately unable to demonstrate wakefulness, and have continuous sleep spindles on EEG. Catecholamine systems therefore seem important in maintaining critical states of wakefulness on the one hand and cortical activation in paradoxical sleep on the other.

As Hobson and McCarley have demonstrated, posterior LC mechanisms are important for the recurrent inhibition of cyclic cholinergic discharges from the pontine FTG, which seem to be responsible for cortical activation in PGO spiking.

Acetylcholine

Acetylcholine and cholinomimetic drugs (physostigmine and pilocarpine) injected into the carotid artery of the rabbit produce arousal, behaviorally and in EEG desynchronization, and activation in the neocortex, hippocampus, caudate nucleus, thalamus, and midbrain reticular system. Arousal reactions to sensory and brainstem reticular stimuli also increase, but these effects can be abolished by the administration of anticholinergic drugs such as atropine. When carbachol, an acetylcholine agonist, is injected into the midbrain near the FTG, the medullary raphe nuclei, or into the fourth ventricle, signs of paradoxical sleep are induced in cats. Destruction of the FTG or interruption of acetylcholine synthesis interrupts not only PGO spikes but the behavioral correlates of paradoxical sleep.

Monnier and Gaillard (1980) noted that cortical slow waves on EEG coexisted with waking behavior when atropine was administered through a carotid cannula. They concluded that atropine caused stronger impairment of cortical structures than subcortical structures. This was interpreted to mean that paradoxical sleep is facilitated by cholinomimetic agents, whereas anticholinergic drugs prevent the dissociation of cortical activity and wakefulness that results in paradoxical sleep.

Sleep-inducing Peptides

Small peptide fractions have recently been found to have several important neurotransmitter or at least regulatory functions as diverse as memory, mood, affect, and pain regulation. A brain protein extracted from sleep-deprived rats induced sleep immediately when injected into the cerebrospinal fluid (CSF) of other rats (Nagasaki, 1974). Later, a small peptide was purified from the spinal fluid of sleep-deprived rats and caused rapid onset of quiet sleep and synchronous EEG slow waves when injected into the ventricles of healthy awake rats (Schoenberger and Monnier, 1977). The active nine-unit peptide, extracted from CSF of sleep-deprived animals or produced synthetically, was capable of inducing delta (slow wave) sleep when injected into the ventricles of several different mammals. It was called delta-sleep-inducing peptide (DSIP) (Monnier and Gaillard, 1980; Kafi, Monnier, and Gaillard, 1979).

Pappenheimer and co-workers found several substances not only in spinal fluid but in plasma and urine of sleep-deprived or sleeping animals (including humans) that were capable of inducing sleep in other mammals (Pappenheimer, 1979; Krueger, Bacsik, and Garcia-Arraras, 1980; Krueger, Pappenheimer, and Karnovsky, 1982). This sleep-promoting small peptide has been found in brain and CSF extracts from goats and rabbits, and also in human plasma and urine. Intraventricular infusion of picomole quantities of this factor is capable of inducing sleep for several hours when administered to rats, rabbits, and cats. The slow wave sleep so produced is normal in that it remains episodic and fluctuating. When the animals are awakened from this stage they are capable of conducting normal behavior; they do not appear narcotized, but are able to awaken normally as from physiological sleep. The purified substance is a small glycopeptide that the Pappenheimer group calls factor S. Two components have been suggested as subunits of factor S, one containing glucosamine and glycine and the other containing glutamine, alanine, diaminopimelic acid, and muramic acid.

Cautious in their interpretation, Pappenheimer et al remain concerned with the distant possibility that factor S could represent a bacterial contaminant. The nonapeptide identified by Monnier and colleagues may be a different compound, requiring 20 μmole per rabbit to induce slow wave sleep, whereas the factor S defined by the Pappenheimer group requires only 10 pmoles to induce the same degree of slow wave sleep. Also, the DSIP of

Monnier only induced 20 to 30 minutes of slow wave sleep, whereas factor S reportedly produces a recurrent pattern of slow wave sleep over a longer period. The concept of protein agents as mediators of sleep may be supported by observations that protein precursors or amino acid loads fed to animals may particularly induce sleep.

Danguir and Nicolaides (1980) and others have failed to induce sleep with putative sleep-inducing peptides (Mendelson, Gillin, and Wyatt, 1981). Using factor S obtained from the Pappenheimer group, Mendelson and associates (1981) were unsuccessful in infusing the peptide into animals. Not only was total sleep time unaffected, but sleep latency was actually prolonged. On balance, however, there is compelling reason to suspect that protein neurotransmitters or neuromodulators play a role at least in the conduction of slow wave sleep, if not other stages. Through metabolism or synthesis of such protein agents, the dietary role in the induction of sleep of certain amino acids such as tryptophan may be explained (Hartmann, 1973).

Benzodiazepine Receptors

Benzodiazepine compounds have emerged as the most widely prescribed group of medications in the world in a very short period of time. Their popularity results from strong sedative and hypnotic properties with generally low toxicity, especially in humans. Such efficacy with low toxicity may imply in itself similarity to intrinsic compounds. Specific protein compounds that preferentially bind benzodiazepines have been identified in several brain areas (Bowling, 1982; Kuhar, 1980). Receptor sites that bind an as yet unrecognized ligand seem to appear late in evolution in humans and apes but not in more primitive mammals. Thus specific benzodiazepine receptors are not apparently a basic neuronal membrane component common to all mammalian systems. Their greatest density is in cerebral cortex, the molecular layer of the cerebellum, in portions of the limbic system, and in the hypothalamus. Although initial reports suggested a neuronal localization of benzodiazepine receptors, there has been some evidence for glial binding sites as well, and even suggestions of preferentially binding in neuronal nuclei. Central benzodiazepine binding sites clearly interact with γ-aminobutyric acid (GABA) recognition (Crawley, 1981). As GABA agonists seem to be primarily inhibitors of neuronal activation, the role of benzodiazepine analogs or receptors in generically inhibitory systems may be of interest. At this point, the role of these receptors in modulating sleep or the sleep-wake cycle remains speculative. Inasmuch as benzodiazepines already are among the most effective inducers of sleep and produce a nearly normal sleep sequence, a role for benzodiazepine receptors in normal sleep regulation is suspected (Tallman, 1980).

Endocrinological Factors

It is important to recognize that sleep functions are components of a broader continuum of behavioral cycles than just the transitions from waking to sleep. During the past 20 years, several fields of biological research which were previously independent have come together with important mutual discoveries. Awareness of biological rhythms, specific physiological phenomena of sleep, and integral control of endocrine functions have become more and more interrelated, to the degree that they must truly be considered a unified field of inquiry (Wagner and Weitzman, 1980).

Claude Bernard's concept of a "constancy of the internal environment" for decades underlay the regulation of endocrine function. Regulation by feedback mechanisms seemed to maintain homeostasis, that is, narrow limits of constancy of hormone secretion. But homeostasis is not always nature's way of regulating endocrine function. Beginning with discoveries of the episodic, pulselike secretion of cortisol, the recognition of discontinuous hormonal secretion became more important. The homeostatic negative feedback control of hormonal function is not applicable to all systems. In 1943 significant daily fluctuation in the secretion of 17-hydroxycorticosteroids (17-OH) was found in the urine of healthy young adults. Much higher amounts are present early in the morning and in the late hours of nocturnal sleep, and very, very small amounts in the later portions of the day. Within ten years it was demonstrated, as expected, that the 17-OH steroids in plasma had a similar cycle. The diurnal fluctuation in this group of steroids was not simply the result of episodic elimination, but apparently was due to episodic production or secretion. In the late 1940s and early 1950s, studies on effects of stress proved that psychological and systemic physiological stress could profoundly alter pituitary function and consequently all known endocrine target glands. Presumably such effects of stress or psychological influence acted through brain and hypothalamic mechanisms, so the revelation that brain activation could influence hypothalamic function became an important topic of endocrinological investigation. With the discovery of a 24-hour cycle in the secretion of 17-OH steroids, interest in other functions with 24-hour cycles grew. It became evident that some systems had briefer oscillations, some of which could be more clearly related to the human 100-minute NREM/REM sleep cycle than to a 24-hour day.

Aristotelian logic probably would predict that endocrinological functions, as mediators of general body activation, metabolism, catabolism, and mood state, must be functionally intertwined with sleep and biological clock organization. If sleep is a state that in part provides protective isolation or at least an adaptive level of activity to climate, light, and temperature variation, then endocrine functions, which regulate reproduction, feeding, body temperature, and body weight, must be attuned to the same temporal cues for successful coping with the environment. If in fact sleep is a biological imperative, but other essential behaviors such as nursing an infant require a cycle shorter than 24 hours, then some endocrine functions would be more effective if episodic lactation and the regulation of hunger in an infant did not have an "environment of constancy," but were periodically and appropriately coordinated with sleep stage or sleep period regulation in infant or mother or both. Hence it should be expected that prolactin (necessary for lactation) and growth hormone (pertinent for infant hunger, metabolism of carbohydrates, and so forth) should be paced by the same timing mechanisms responsible for sleep sequences. By contrast, hormones such as cortisol that particularly influence responsiveness to the stresses of climate or external environment should more nearly be pegged to a 24-hour cycle, so that a peak secretion of adrenocorticotropic hormone (ACTH) and subsequently of 17-OH steroids might prepare the human for feeding, foraging, hunting, or conflict with the coming of dawn in preparation for daytime activities.

Pituitary-Hypothalamic Factors

Current evidence suggests that the anterior pituitary hormones as a group—ACTH, growth hormone (GH), prolactin (PRL), thyroid-stimulating hormone (TSH), and luteinizing hormone (LH)—are secreted in a pulsatile manner, each with its own relationship to some aspect of the sleep-wake cycle, 24-hour calendar or climate variability, or the REM/NREM cycle. They are regulated by a combination of open-loop control mechanisms mediated largely by releasing or inhibiting factors from the hypothalamus and, in the cases of at least ACTH, TSH, FSH, and LH, also a mediating closed-loop negative feedback response to circulating levels of a target hormone. Hypothalamic pathways responsible for these anterior pituitary hormones may be proximally mediated by norepinephrine, dopamine, or serotonin, among the neurotransmitters that control sleep mechanisms. The mechanisms responsible for sleep-related individual hormonal secretion conceivably could differ from those that cause response of the same target hormone tested in the waking state. For some of the anterior pituitary hormones, the effects of sleep seem to vary with age or level of development. This may be especially pertinent for growth hormone and gonadotropins. In some cases, such as luteinizing hormone and cortisol, the relationship to the sleep-wake cycle persists even in diseases characterized by oversecretion of the hormone.

Melatonin, found not only in anterior pituitary but in the pineal gland, may play a role, as yet undefined, in regulation of sleep sequence and perhaps effect one of the feedback-mediating influences on pituitary regulation.

To demonstrate a relationship between the sleep-wake cycle and hormonal secretion, and especially to demonstrate a relationship with specific sleep stages, there are two important requirements:

1. It must be possible to detect rapid changes in plasma concentration of a hormone because of episodic secretion and short plasma half-life of some hormones, whether due to consumption or distribution.
2. It is necessary to recognize and contend with rapid changes of sleep stages if any influence between various sleep stages and the hormones in question is to be clarified.

For most hormones, satisfying these two requirements necessitates plasma samples taken at least every 15 to 20 minutes for no less than 24 hours. Less frequent sampling may give rise to errors by missing changes in sleep cycle or failing to detect fluctuating concentrations of various hormones (Quabe, 1978).

With greater recognition of hypothalamic cell populations in sleep regulation, the substrate for interaction of hypothalamic-pituitary regulation and sleep-wake regulation begins to emerge. Sleep-inducing peptides have some chemical similarities to neuropeptides responsible for pituitary stimulation. Catecholamines and indoleamines are important for sleep induction and sleep sequencing as well as for diffuse endocrinological functions. In addition to the biochemical similarities, sleep functions and endocrine regulation also share common anatomical territory. The sleep-wake cycle and endocrine regulation are obviously closely related components of the same biological behavioral adaptive system.

Recognizing that some hormonal systems are based on a 24-hour clock but others depend instead on sleeping-waking rhythms may have very practical implications. Clarifying biological rhythms may provide insights into several important common clinical syndromes, including acromegaly, Cushing's syndrome, and probably depression and bipolar depressive disease. Similarly, as synthetic hormones become more widely available and as nucleic acid manipulations may provide complex hormonal substitutes not currently available for clinical use, the appropriate administration of such substances might hinge upon understanding the temporal sequence of hormone function in nature.

ACTH and Cortisol

Pulsatile secretion of hormones was first recognized in reproducible diurnal rhythm in the excretion of urinary ketosteroids by young male Army inductees in the 1940's (Pincus, 1943). Although the intervals and collection of some urine specimens were somewhat imprecise, it was possible to show definitively that there was a much higher concentration and a much higher total secretion of ketosteroids in the daytime hours than at night, and most especially in urine collected in the morning. Even subjects with higher concentrations than average at night still had much higher concentrations in their morning urine ketosteroids. A few subjects were taken from emergency calls in hospital and these were associated with higher steroid secretion, but even in the face of stress, morning secretion was higher than that during the night.

In the ensuing 20 years, it became clear that not only urinary products of corticosteroids were increased in the morning, but actually the secretions seemed to be highest in the early hours even before awakening. Halberg et al (1961) showed that even among subjects totally deprived of sleep for one or two nights, episodic secretion of cortisol in the early morning hours continued despite lack of sleep. In other words, the cortisol cycle did not require sleep in order to peak at early morning hours.

Using a small indwelling catheter in an arm vein of sleeping healthy volunteers, and simultaneously monitoring sleep stages with EEG, it became possible to draw frequent small samples of plasma for determination of corticosteroids and thus be more precise about pattern times of release of hormones (Weitzman, Schaumburg, Fishbein, 1966, and Weitzman, de Graff, and Sassin, 1975). Studying cortisol secretion in this manner, two or three major peaks in the early morning hours were recorded. Since these peaks had approximately a 60- to 90-minute cycle in several cases, Weitzman and colleagues concluded that there was a link between cortisol or ACTH secretion and REM sleep. They noted that the bulk of REM sleep occurred in the latter half of the night, and was particularly more intense and longer in duration in the few hours before awakening. Since the REM cycle had about a 90-minute interval, this seemed to be appropriate for the two peaks noted. When the sleep-wake cycle was inverted and the sleep occurred in daytime, however, the major peak of cortisol secretion continued in the very early hours in the morning; and with more frequent intervals, sometimes the multiple peak secretions were not found. Extending the studies to 24-hour basis, these investigators found that episodic cortisol secretion did indeed persist throughout that period, but the clustering of greatest secretory episodes was still in the early hours of morning. They emphasized that there was no "basal level or steady state" of secretion for any extended period of time during the 24 hours, but truly an episodic pulsatile type of secretion throughout the day with clear maximum secretion early in the morning, whether or not the subject was asleep.

The cortisol secretory phase is not altogether independent of the sleep cycle. When healthy volunteers were entrained to a three-hour day with two hours awake and one hour asleep for prolonged periods, a cycle with maximum secretion anticipating the next awakening phase could be produced. Still, the peak at these times was not as high as that when the subject was entrained to a typical 24-hour sleep-wake day. Also, a superimposed 24-

hour pattern did continue; despite eight recurring cycles of 3-hour days in every 24-hour period, there was still a maximum secretion of both ACTH and cortisol between the hours of 4 and 6 AM (Wagner and Weitzman, 1980). This demonstrates not only the stability of the underlying ACTH secretory phase but that the ACTH/cortisol axis does adapt to sleep cycle shifts to some degree. Such responsiveness of ACTH secretion is very conservative, of course, maintaining the supervening pattern built around a 24-hour cycle. In similar studies, Weitzman reported measuring 24-hour plasma cortisol secretions in healthy subjects from an arctic environment where there are enormous differences during the year in the daily ratio of sunlight and dark. Although there was a very slight increase in mean plasma concentration and total amount of cortisol secreted over 24-hour periods in the autumn and winter (presumably related to greater metabolic stress), there was no difference in circadian pattern of secretion. Weitzman concluded that although social and work schedules may be influential, the direct influence of environment in terms of sleeping and waking cues and light and darkness did not alter secretion.

Diurnal cycles of cortisol secretion may persist, even if altered, in disease states. Patients with Cushing's syndrome may continue a diurnal secretion of the cortisol hormone even as an exaggeration of the normal episodic pattern. This may depend on whether the hypersecretion is due to increased amount of ACTH and cortisol-releasing factor or due to an adrenal cortical adenoma. Patients with Cushing's syndrome resulting from hypothalamic excess have an exaggerated 24-hour cyclic peak, whereas those with adrenal adenomas have been reported to have continuously elevated secretion of cortisol, either not fluctuating significantly or failing to maintain a reproducible diurnal schedule.

Aldosterone and corticosterone follow an episodic early morning secretion similar to that of cortisol, even in the face of sodium restriction.

The adaptive benefits of secreting the hormones needed to cope with stress and to prepare for the hunt just before awakening are obvious. The mechanism for coordinating diurnal cyclic hormonal secretion with a 24-hour bed and arousal schedule may be that the same hypothalamic nuclei perform both functions, or at least the nuclei responsible for both functions are anatomically close. Anatomically, corticotropin-releasing factor (CRF) and ACTH are both compounds derived from paraventricular hypothalamic nuclei or nearby structures. That is, they are secreted and regulated by cell groups near the supraoptic and suprachiasmatic nuclei, which are keys in initiating early phases of sleep. Whether or not direct neuronal synapses of humoral mediating substances are responsible for coordination of sleep function and endocrine systems remains speculative, but proximity of important regulating centers is apparent.

The regularity of the ACTH cycle is strong enough to be resistant to changes in sleep-wake patterns on short terms. Up to 205 hours of sleep deprivation or significant changes in the total amount of sleep for one or two days at a time does not significantly alter either the amount or the timing of an ACTH or cortisol secretory peak (Mendelson, Gillin, and Wyatt, 1977).

Some reports have suggested that patients with anorexia nervosa lack a 24-hour secretory pattern for ACTH. This has been a controversial topic, because several patients with florid anorexia nervosa have demonstrated clear-cut 24-hour pulsatile secretions of ACTH, sometimes with near-normal overall ACTH secretion (Weitzman, de Graff, and Sassin, 1975). Perhaps this is a clinical syndrome with more than one biological basis, with some cases accompanied by an abnormal sleep-wake pattern of cortisol secretion and others maintaining normal secretory phases.

Wagner and Weitzman (1980) pointed out that Cushing's disease is characterized not only by abnormal ACTH-cortisol rhythms, but by psychiatric disorders, most especially serious mood disorders of which depression is the most evident. They noted also that patients with Addison's disease frequently are depressed and also lack the normal periodicity of ACTH secretion. Patients with endogenous as opposed to reactive or "neurotic" depression seem to lack the normal circadian rhythmical control of cortisol that occurs in patients with Cushing's disease. In fact, cortisol secretions in such chronically depressed people may reach levels often seen among patients with Cushing's disease. When one considers these disturbances in ACTH secretion and rhythmical control as well as the reversal of normal circadian rhythm patterns, and the observation that manipulation of sleep cycles, particularly increased amounts of REM sleep, may be seen among persons with endogenous depression, the relative interaction of endocrine functions, sleep-wake cycles, and affective disorders or mood regulation becomes more complicated. What is clear is that the three systems do interact in a complex manner, so that it is impossible biologically to separate them.

The corticotropin-releasing factor (CRF)/ACTH axis seems to be under the stimulating influence of serotonin (5HT) and to be inhibited by norepinephrine. If in fact norepinephrine is a neurotransmitter that is deficient in the genesis of depression, the CRF/ACTH/cortisol axis may be integrally related to the REM cycle only as a mutual effect of serotonin secretion or by the absence of norepinephrine release. As Wagner and Weitzman (1980) point out, it is possible that the disturbed rhythm of ACTH and cortisol release in depressed persons may be an epiphenomenon or byproduct of the depression, or may just as likely reflect a disordered limbic-hypothalamic interrelationship. At any rate, the disturbance of cortisol and ACTH rhythmicity and response to pharmacological agents such as dexamethasone suppression may be useful for diagnosing different forms of depression, the effects of therapy, and the effect of endocrine dependence upon sleep-wake cycles.

Growth Hormone

Growth hormone (GH) is the first substance found responsive to a particular phase of sleep, not just sleep onset. It is particularly linked to slow wave sleep stages III and IV (Sassin, Parker, and Mace, 1969; Weitzman, de Graff, and Sassin, 1975). The relationship between sleep onset and growth hormone release is intriguing. Jacoby et al (1974) demonstrated that intravenous injections of monoamine precursors induced the concurrent onset of slow wave sleep and marked secretion of growth hormone in monkeys. 5-Hydroxytryptophan induced behavioral sleep and EEG slow wave sleep, but serotonin was able to induce a more rapid onset of sleep and higher elevations in growth hormone. Intravenous infusion of glucose, however, which at other times may interfere with growth hormone secretion, did not prevent the increase in growth hormone secretion associated with slow wave sleep. Slow wave sleep alone is not sufficient to induce growth hormone release; during slow wave sleep in the second half of the night, there may be no detectable GH secretion, or only trivial amounts.

Puig-Antich, et al (1978) suggested that deprivation of slow wave sleep in childhood may interfere with release of growth hormone and could cause delay or retardation in growth (so-called biosocial dwarfs). An interesting observation is that children with constitutionally short stature may have normal GH responses to insulin injection (a standard for determining normal GH responsiveness). They also have normal sleep-related growth hormone peaks. By contrast, patients with short stature caused by hypopituitarism (whether idiopathic or due to hypothalamic mass lesions) usually have diminished secretion of growth hormone in response to insulin injection, and also diminished secretion in early slow wave sleep at night.

It is not just early "deep" sleep that is necessary for the secretion of GH. Deprivation of early slow wave sleep reliably lowers GH secretion, but selective REM deprivation does not have this effect. Quabe (1978) noted that slow wave sleep may be present for as long as 60 minutes before GH is secreted or detected, and also that during slow wave sleep epochs late in the night there is seldom a GH peak. These and other observations led Quabe to conclude that slow wave sleep and nocturnal-release GH may result from a common releasing mechanism, rather than GH being a direct cause and effect on slow wave sleep. This was suggested also by the studies of Jacoby et al who showed that monoamines capable of inducing slow wave sleep were able to induce growth hormone release as well (1974).

Since hypothyroidism has been reported occasionally to cause increased amounts of slow wave sleep, Mendelson, Gillin, and Wyatt (1977) speculated whether hyperthyroidism might similarly lead to an increased secretion of growth hormone. They reported two patients with hypothyroidism who, with increased duration of slow wave sleep, had elevations in levels of plasma GH. After treatment, slow wave sleep returned to 20 percent of the total sleep time and GH secretion diminished.

Effects of sleep on growth hormone may be very important in regard to wound healing following operations or injury and recovery from tissue destruction seen with myocardial or cerebral infarction and pulmonary emboli. If deprivation of slow wave sleep, particularly in the early phases of sleep, impairs GH release, the effects upon fibroblasts, significantly influenced by GH for wound healing and metabolism, may be to impair healing. As discussed by Orr (Chapter 7), the environment in recovery rooms, hospital services, and intensive care units may significantly alter sleeping patterns, which influence not only the emotional state of the patient, but biological recovery.

The daily pattern of GH secretion, of course, varies with age. The neonate secretes high levels in a rather random manner throughout the day, irrespective of sleep-wake cycles. Of course, the neonate sleeps for up to 18 hours of a 24-hour cycle, and particularly in the first few weeks the sequence is chaotic. As a circadian pattern of sleep-wake regulation develops at approximately 16 weeks postpartum, or after the sixtieth gestational week, secretory patterns of GH begin to assume a regular cycle. Only near the age of 9 or 10 years, in the prepubertal stage, do children begin to show the clear sleep-related release of growth hormone. As slow wave sleep has been related to daytime levels of activity, so also is secretion of GH. When four children were treated with complete bedrest, they had no waking state secretion of GH, but when allowed to ambulate and be active, there was at least some low level of secretion (Finkelstein, Roffwarg, Boyar, et al, 1972). Of course the highest concentrations during slow wave sleep of any age group are seen among adolescent or puberty-aged children, and even among this age group there may also be smaller daytime secretion bursts one to four times throughout the day. This increase occurs not only during the growth bursts of early adolescence, but is seen among young adults who generally have higher levels of GH than prepubertal children. By the age of 50 years, it falls to virtually undetectable levels even throughout sleep. It is of interest to speculate whether this is simply the result of diminished slow wave sleep, or whether both the slow wave sleep and the diminished secretion of GH are products of diminished hypothalamic dopamine activity.

Acromegaly, a disease characterized by increased secretions of growth hormone, provides a model both for studying the endocrine system and coupling the endocrine secretion with sleep regulation. The disease results from an adenoma that secretes growth hormone in excessive amounts, generally throughout the 24-hour day, although there is occasionally peak secretion during nocturnal, early slow wave sleep. If the disease begins during childhood before the epiphyses of long bones close, it leads to extreme height, the so-called pituitary giant. More commonly, however, the disease begins after the epiphyses close. This causes growth of distal or acral parts, such as the hands, fingers, feet, and mandible. The results are coarse facial features, joint diseases, and cardiomegaly. Glucose intolerance (diabetes) is the product of growth hormone and insulin interaction. There may be two major forms of acromegaly, distinguished by the response of GH secretion to thyrotropin-releasing hormone (TRH) or to L-dopa (a natural inhibitor of GH) and bromocriptine (an ergot compound with dopaminergic properties). In some patients with acromegaly who have GH release in response to TRH, L-dopa is able to suppress growth hormone. Those who do not respond to TRH do not show suppression of GH in response to L-dopa. Bromocriptine, now commercially available, behaves the same as L-dopa in either form of acromegaly. Wagner and Weitzman (1980) concluded that the differential responsiveness to bromocriptine/L-dopa or TRH probably represents different sensitivity among tumor cell receptors rather than totally different hypothalamic or pituitary mechanisms of the disease.

Whereas most adults have undetectable levels of GH during daytime, in persons with acromegaly levels virtually never drop so far as to be undetectable. Other pituitary hormones or pituitary-regulated hormones affect the secretion of GH. Somatostatin has been shown to impair its physiological release, but the effect of such inhibition is constant in either the waking or sleep stage, and the infusion of somatostatin or influence of somatotropin-release-inhibiting factor (SRIF) seems unaffected by sleep-waking cycle or sleep stage at the time of injection (Parker, Rossman, and Siler, 1974). In males, the early prepubertal increase in GH release is affected by plasma testosterone, but the response of GH to high levels of testosterone and the sequence of testosterone and GH secretion seem independent of nocturnal sleep stage patterns (Thompson, Rodriguez, and Kowarski, 1972).

Growth hormone may be a factor in regulation of sleep sequences, perhaps through feedback on the suprachiasmatic nucleus, or on other neuroendocrine functions. In rats, GH caused longer and more intense paradoxical sleep (Drucker-Colin, Spanis, Hunyadi, et al, 1975; Stern, Jalowiec, Shabshelowitz, et al, 1975) and in fact, the injection of GH in sleeping mice may actually influence memory or memory functions upon later awakening. Working with healthy human volunteers in a crossover study, Mendelson et al (1980) found that the injection of 2 units of growth hormone intramuscularly 15 minutes before bedtime had no measurable effect on sleep functions as determined by EEG. When 5 units were injected instead of 2, however, there was a 19 percent decrement of slow wave sleep and 13 percent increase in REM sleep. Neither dose when given during daytime hours affected tests of learning in the subjects or induced sleep. In a study of the effects of intravenous injections of several monoamine precursors and of apomorphine (an L-dopa agonist) in monkeys, it was found that both L-dopa (in concentrations of 15 to 200 mg per kg) and serotonin (20 to 60 mg per kg) were able to induce an acute elevation in plasma GH concentration. Neither induced hypoglycemia, so the release of GH was induced by a direct central nervous system function, and was not a response to hypoglycemia (Jacoby, Smith, and Sassin, 1975).

When tryptophan, the immediate precursor of serotonin, was administered to young adults in doses of 50 to 100 mg per kg, it induced a smaller elevation of growth hormone after a brief lag but simultaneously with onset of slow wave sleep. Growth hormone secretion may be elicited by intravenous injection of L-dopa, but usually without associated slow wave sleep. Apomorphine does not induce GH release during sleep in humans. From these conclusions, it would appear that while GH may be induced or released by several monoamines, often concurrently with slow wave sleep, there are probably independent mechanisms that may respond at times to common neurotransmitters. In the efficiency of biological conservation, it is reasonable to expect that certain monoamines such as serotonin might be used by the organism for synchronizing onset of several cyclic behaviors, such as hormones on one hand and sleep stages on the other.

Thyroid-Stimulating Hormone

For many years the thyroid/pituitary axis seemed to be the very paradigm of the closed-loop negative feedback model of classic endocrine homeostasis. The active forms of thyroid hormone, triiodothyronine (T_3) and tetraiodothyronine (T_4), are both secreted by the thyroid in response to thyroid-stimulating hormone (TSH), an anterior pituitary hormone. Characterization of the diurnal sequence of TSH release has been confounded in the past by two factors: the lack of a sensitive assay for low concentrations, and until recently, the lack of a hypothalamic releasing factor for TSH. When the tightly coupled association between TSH and the thyroid hormones was considered, any variability of TSH during the daytime was generally considered to be an artifact of the measuring technique in the small quantities of hormone present (Wagner and Weitzman, 1980; Peters, Santa-Cruz, Tower, et al, 1981).

Earliest studies of a diurnal sequence of TSH secretion suggested a peak well after sleep onset, but such studies were hampered by the failure to record sleep polygraphically, hence sleep sequence was not rigidly defined. More recent studies have consistently shown that TSH levels rise in the two to four hours prior to onset of sleep. Often secretion begins to fall either with onset of sleep or shortly afterward (Wagner and Weitzman, 1980; Parker, Pekary, and Hershman, 1976). Since total T_4 and T_3 vary only minimally throughout the day, and even then only in response to posture, activity, or emotion, the diurnal variability of circulating TSH is perplexing. It should be recognized that thyroid-releasing hormone (TRH) is less a releasing transmitter than a modulator. Peters et al (1981) showed that TRH infusion significantly elevated levels of serum TSH over baseline controls when injected during slow wave sleep and REM sleep, more during slow wave sleep. As Oswald (1980) points out, the apparent anabolic function of several phases of sleep may depend upon functions of TSH that are as yet unidentified. That is, the combined actions of TSH and GH together may influence other anabolic functions during sleep that are unrelated to effects exerted only upon the thyroid.

Prolactin

Unlike the other pituitary hormones, prolactin seems to be primarily regulated by an inhibitory modulator rather than a prolactin-releasing factor, and the prolactin-inhibitory factor (PIF) seems to be not only dopaminergic, but may in fact be dopamine itself. Additionally, prolactin itself may have a feedback inhibition such that high levels of serum prolactin may in the healthy state inhibit further prolactin secretion. Among the physiological states that cause transient elevation of prolactin levels are hypoglycemia, significant physical exercise, severe physical stress, or moderate degrees of psychic stress. Suckling in postpartum women, or even significant breast manipulation as in sexual foreplay, increases prolactin concentrations in adult women. Although TRH does induce a slight rise in serum prolactin, it does not appear to be a significant physiological prolactin-releasing factor (Wagner and Weitzman, 1980).

In the individual with a single nocturnal sleep period, prolactin secretion precedes the release of serum cortisol by two to three hours and the two peak simultaneously just at or before awakening. This fact suggested that prolactin, like cortisol, was tied to a 24-hour cycle and not to sleep events of the night. Subsequent studies of the association of prolactin with fragmented sleep periods or daytime naps show that prolactin release is tied directly to sleep behavior. Daytime naps clearly induce a sharp elevation in levels of serum prolactin, and the link seems to be caused by sleep per se rather than time of day or even to particular phases of sleep. Unlike growth hormone, serum prolactin secretion is neither directly tied to nor accelerated or intensified by deprivation of slow wave sleep. Even among prepubertal children of either sex, levels increase with sleep. Sleep-related fluctuations in levels seem to persist even past menopause. Even when levels of serum prolactin increase with those of luteinizing hormone in midovulation, the highest levels of serum prolactin occur in sleep.

Serum prolactin secretion is increased in several hypothalamic and pituitary diseases because the primary regulatory hormone is an inhibitory factor. Disease of the hypothalamus lowers this inhibitory factor and allows excessive secretion of prolactin. The sleep-wake rhythm of prolactin secretion is either blunted or absent in Cushing's disease, drug-induced hyperprolactinemia, or even in so-called primary prolactinomas. High levels of the hormone in these states seem to persist either in the waking or sleeping states (Wagner and Weitzman, 1980).

The clearest physiological function of the hormone prolactin is to induce or permit lactation. Inasmuch as a symbiotic coordination of synchronization of the sleeping patterns between mother and infant would seem to be efficient in order to coordinate effective sleep for both parties, a good method would be to link lactation and milk storage to those times when the mother is able to rest comfortably and prepare for feeding shortly after awakening. A selective advantage to coordinating prolactin release and subsequent milk synthesis during sleep, even short (nap) periods, seems reasonably obvious.

SUMMARY

The sleep process is clearly more than just a respite from daytime activity. Rather, sleep provides an intricate, and at present puzzling, change in many physiological functions. To be sure, some of them appear to have *restorative* (and hence "resting") functions, but others involve complex endocrine changes that obviously impact on all other body systems.

Little imagination is required to see that many features of human behavior are intertwined with the regulation of sleep.

REFERENCES

Battini C, Magni F, Paletini M, Rossi G, Zanchetti M. Neuronal mechanisms underlying EEG and behavioral activation in the midpontine pretrigeminal cat. Arch Ital Biol 1959;13–25.

Bowling B. Micromolar affinity of benzodiazepine receptors: identification and characterization in central nervous system. Science 1982;216:1247–50.

Brodal A. The reticular formation of the brain stem. Anatomical aspects and functional correlations. Edinburgh: Oliver & Boyd, 1957.

Cajal R. Histologie du système nerveux. Vol. I. Madrid: Consejo superior de investigaciones científicas, 1952.

Clemente C. Cortical synchronization and the onset of sleep. In: Kales A, ed. Sleep: physiology and pathology. Philadelphia: JB Lippincott, 1969.

Clemente C, Sterman S, Wyrwicka W. Forebrain inhibitory mechanisms: conditioning of basal forebrain induced EEG synchronization and sleep. Exp Neurol 1963;7:404.

Crawley J. Neuropharmacologic specificity of a simple animal model for the behavioral actions of benzodiazepines. Pharmacol Biochem Behav 1981;15:695–99.

Danguir J, Nicolaides S. Intravenous infusions of nutrients and sleep in the rat: an ischymetric sleep regulation hypothesis. Am J Physiol 1980;238(4):E307–12.

Drucker-Colin R, Spanis C, Hunyadi J, Sassin J, McGaugh J. Growth hormone effects on sleep and wakefulness in the rat. Neuroendocrinology 1975;18:1.

Finkelstein J, Roffwarg H, Boyar R, Kream J, Hellman L. Age-related change in the twenty-four-hour spontaneous secretion of growth hormone. J Clin Endocrinol Metabol 1972;35:665–70.

Fulton J, Ingraham F. Emotional disturbances following experimental lesions of the base of the brain (prechiasmal). J Physiol (London) 1929;67:27.

Halberg F, Frank G, Harner R, et al. The adrenal cycle in men on different schedules of motor and mental activity. Experientia 1961;17:282–84.

Hartmann E. The functions of sleep. New Haven: Yale University Press, 1973.

Hobson JA, McCarley R. The brain as a dream state generator: an activation-synthesis hypothesis of the dream process. Am J Psychiatry 1977;134:1335–48.

Hobson JA, McCarley RW, Freedman R. Time course of discharge rate changes by cat pontine stem neurons in desynchronized sleep. J Neurophysiol 1974;371:1297–1309.

Hobson JA, McCarley RW, Freedman R, Pivik R. Selective firing by cat pontine brain stem neurons in desynchronized sleep. J Neurophysiol 1974;37:497–511.

Hobson JA, McCarley RW, Wyzinski P. Sleep cycle oscillation: reciprocal discharge by two brainstem neuronal groups. Science 1975;189:55–8.

Jacoby JH, Sassin JF, Greenstein M. Patterns of spontaneous cortisol and growth hormone secretion in rhesus monkeys during the sleep-waking cycle. Neuroendocrinology 1974;14:165–73.

Jacoby J, Smith E, Sassin J. Altered growth hormone secretory pattern following prolonged sleep deprivation in the monkey. Neuroendocrinology 1975;18:9–15.

Jeannerod M, Mouret J, Jouvet M. Effets secondaires de la déafferentation visuelle sur l'activité phasique pontogeniculo-occipitale du sommeil paradoxal. J Physiol (Paris) 1965;57:255.

Jouvet M. Recherches sur les structures nerveuses et les mécanismes responsables des différentes phases du sommeil physiologique. Arch Ital Biol 1962;100:125–206.

Jouvet M. Mechanisms of the states of sleep. A neuropharmacological approach. Res Publ Assoc Res Nerv Ment Dis 1967a;45:86–126.

Jouvet M. Neurophysiology of the states of sleep. Physiol Rev 1967b;47:117.

Jouvet M. Neurophysiological and biochemical mechanisms of sleep. In: Kales A, ed. Sleep: physiology and pathology. Philadelphia: JB Lippincott, 1969.

Jouvet M, Delorme F. Organisation du systéme responsable de l'activite phasique au cours du sommeil paradoxal. C.R. Soc Biol 1965;159:1599–1604.

Kafi S, Monnier M, Gaillard JM. The delta-sleep-inducing peptide (DSIP) increases duration of sleep in rats. Neurosci Lett 1979;13:164–72.

Koella WP. Sleep, its nature and physiological origin. Springfield, Ill.: Charles C Thomas, 1967.

Krueger JM, Bacsik J, Garcia-Arraras J. Sleep-promoting material from human urine and its relation to factor S from brain. Am J Physiol 1980;238:E116–23.

Krueger JM, Pappenheimer JR, Karnovsky ML. The composition of sleep-promoting factor isolated from human urine. J Biol Chem 1982;257:1664–69.

Kuhar M. The benzodiazepine receptor: anatomical aspects. NIDA Research Monogram Series 1980;33:12–21.

Lydic R, Schoene WC, Czeisler CA, Moore-Ede MC. Suprachiasmatic region of the human hypothalamus: homolog to the primate circadian pacemaker? Sleep 1980;2:355–61.

McCarley RW. REM sleep dreams, and the activation-synthesis hypothesis. Am J Psychiatry 1981;138:904–12.

McCarley RW, Hobson JA. Neuronal excitability modulation over the sleep cycle: a structural and mathematical model. Science 1975;189:58–60.

Mendelson WB, Gillin JC, Wyatt RJ. Human sleep and its disorders. New York: Plenum Press, 1977.

Mendelson WB, Gillin JC, Wyatt RJ. Where is the hypnotoxin? Presented at the twenty-first annual meeting of the Association for the Psychophysiological Study of Sleep, Hyannis, Massachusetts, June 1981.

Mendelson WB, Slater S, Gold P, Gillin JC. The effect of growth hormone administration on human sleep: a dose-response study. Biol Psychiatry 1980;15:613–18.

Monnier M, Gaillard J. Biochemical regulation of sleep. Experientia 1980;36:21–24.

Moore RY. The anatomy of central neural mechanisms regulating endocrine rhythms. In: Krieger DT, ed. Endocrine rhythms. New York: Raven Press, 1979:63–68.

Moore RY, Eichler V. Central neural mechanism in diurnal rhythm regulation and neuroendocrine response to light. Psychoneuroendocrinology 1976;1:265–79.

Moruzzi G, Magoun H. Brainstem reticular formation and activation of the EEG. Electroencephalogr Clin Neurophysiol 1949;1:455–73.

Nagasaki H. The presence of sleep-promoting material in the brain of sleep-deprived rats. Proc Jpn Acad Sci 1974;50:241–46.

Nauta W. Hypothalamic regulation of sleep in rats. J Neurophysiol 1946;9:285.

Oswald I. Sleep as a restorative process: human clues. Prog Brain Res 1980;53:279–88.

Pappenheimer J. Factor S, a sleep-promoting protein in human urine. Johns Hopkins Med J 1979;145:49–56.

Parker D, Pekary A, Hershman J. Effect of normal and revised sleep-wake cycles upon nyctohemeral rhythmicity of plasma thyrotropin: evidence suggestive of an inhibiting influence of sleep. J Clin Endocrinol Metab 1976;43:318–29.

Parker DC, Rossman LG, Siler TM. Inhibition of the sleep-related peak in physiologic human growth hormone release by somatostatin. J Clin Endocrinol Metab 1974;38:496–9.

Peters J, Santa-Cruz F, Tower B, Rubin R. Differential neuroendocrine responses to thyrotropin-releasing hormone during rapid eye movement and slow wave sleep in man. J Clin Endocrinol Metab 1981;52:975–81.

Pincus, G. Diurnal rhythm in excretion of urine ketosteroids by young men. J Clin Endocrinology 1943;3:195–199.

Pompeiano O. The neurophysiological mechanisms of the postural and motor events during desynchronized sleep. Res Publ Assoc Res Nerv Ment Dis 1967;45:351–423.

Puig-Antich J, Greenhill LL, Sassin J, Sachar EJ. Growth hormone, prolactin and cortisol responses and growth patterns in hyperkinetic children treated with dextro-amphetamine. Preliminary findings. J Am Acad Child Psychiatry 1978;17:457–75.

Quabe H. Endocrine concomitants of the sleep-wake cycle in man. In: Assenmacher I, Farner D, eds. Environmental Endocrinology. Berlin: Springer Verlag, 1978:124–31.

Roffwarg H, Dement W, Muzio J. Dream imagery: relationship to rapid eye movements of sleep. Arch Gen Psychiatry 1962;7:235–8.

Rusak B, Zucker I. Neural regulation of circadian rhythms. Physiol Rev 1979;59:449–526.

Sassin JF, Parker DC, Mace JW. Human growth hormone release: relation to slow-wave sleep and sleep-walking cycles. Science 1969;165:513–5.

Scheibel J, Scheibel A. Anatomical basis of attention mechanisms in vertebrate brains. In: Quarton G, Melnechuk T, Schmitt F, eds. The neurosciences: a study program. New York: Rockefeller University Press, 1967:577–602.

Schoenberger G, Monnier M. Characterization of the delta EEG sleep inducing peptide. Proc Natl Acad Sci USA 1977;74:1282–86.

Schwartz W, Gainer H. Localization of the "biological clock" in the brain. JAMA 1981;246:681.

Shagass C, Trusty D. Somatosensory and visual cerebral evoked responses changes during sleep. In: Wortis J, ed. Recent advances in biological psychiatry. New York: Plenum Press, 1967.

Stern W, Jalowiec J, Shabshelowitz H, Morgane P. Effects of growth hormone on sleep-waking patterns in cats. Horm Behav 1975;6:189–196.

Tallman J. Benzodiazepines: biochemistry and function. NIDA Research Monograph series 1980;33:4–12.

Thompson RG, Rodriguez A, Kowarski A. Integrated concentrations of growth hormone correlated with plasma testosterone and bone age in preadolescent and adolescent males. Endocrinology 1972;35:334–7.

Wagner D, Weitzman E. Neuroendocrine secretion and biological rhythms in man. Psychiatr Clin North Am 1980;3:223–50.

Weitzman ED, deGraff AS, Sassin JF. Seasonal patterns of sleep stages and secretion of cortisol and growth hormone during 24 hour period in northern Norway. Acta Endocrinol (Kbh) 1975;78(1):65–76.

Weitzman ED, Schaumburg H, Fishbein W. Plasma 17-hydroxycorticosteroid levels during sleep in man. J Clin Endocrinol 1966;26:121–7.

Yamazaki I, Ishikawa T, Nakamura M, Yokota K-N, Nakamura S. Metabolic oscillations in homogeneous and heterogeneous systems. In: Suda M., Hayaishi O, Nakagawa, H., eds. Biologic rhythms and their central mechanism. North Holland: Elsevier. 1979:19–28.

CHAPTER 3

Behavioral Aspects of Sleep
Terrence L. Riley and
Richard Ferber

The basic human need for sleep varies greatly, ranging between 4 and 10 hours among healthy individuals. Normally short sleepers tend to be very active, but attempt to be productive and are often deemed well adjusted by their contemporaries (Hartmann, Baekeland, and Zwilling, 1972). By contrast, those who generally sleep 10 hours or more a day tend to be more relaxed or phlegmatic, often are perceived as low keyed by contemporaries, frequently appear mildly depressed, and sometimes are characterized as underachievers (Hartmann, Baekeland, and Zwilling, 1972). Of course, there are many exceptions to the generalizations. Albert Einstein, for example, often would sleep for 14 to 16 hours for many consecutive days. Certainly, he was a very reflective and outwardly relaxed individual, but just as clearly he was productive and well reconciled to his environment. Long or short sleeping habits often seem to be familial traits. Genetically controlled experiments among animals have shown marked strain differences in sleep length, most notable in rodents and also in other mammalian strains (Valatx and Bugat, 1974). Among humans, of course, it is difficult to know the degree to which such traits might be inherited or acquired. Both long and short sleepers seem to have rather constant amounts of slow wave sleep at given ages, although long sleepers tend to have much more rapid eye movement (REM) sleep (Hartmann, Baekeland, and Zwilling, 1972; Williams, Karacan, and Hursch, 1974). Meddis, Pearson, and Langford (1973) reported a 70-year-old woman who slept only 67 minutes per night and claimed to have maintained such a short sleeping period all her life. In fact, when asked about her sleeping habits she was surprised to learn that other people need more sleep. When she was studied at the sleep laboratory, 16.5 percent of total sleep time was REM, 32.6 percent slow wave sleep, and 50 percent stage II sleep (Meddis, Pearson, and Langford, 1973). In her case, the relative proportions of most of the sleep stages seemed to be the same as in people with normal sleep duration. Other examples of persons with dramatically short sleep patterns have been demonstrated, and when brief total times have been found, normal percentages of the stages have been reported (Mendelson, Gillin, and Wyatt, 1977).

As REM sleep has been the most conspicuous focus of attention in sleep research, it is not surprising that the behavior during this stage has been of concern. The functions of REM sleep have often centered on cognition and learning. In a study of memory and learning during sleep, short-term memory or recall for simple events such as brief sounds, tactile stimuli, and short words was shown to be possible in most stages of sleep, although less accurate in slow wave sleep (Cohen, 1980). Novel or complex stimuli evoked higher-frequency patterns in the electroencephalogram (EEG) of the sleeping individual than in the waking EEG. It seems possible that some complex stimuli may be processed in REM sleep, but are lost with awakening. Recall of complex verbal information seems to be dependent upon EEG activation, that is, desynchronization and lowering of voltage. If the stimulus or item to be learned or recalled is not delivered in such a manner that EEG activation or high-frequency response occurs, then it is not likely that such information will be recalled either awake or asleep, as though there were a gate between short- and long-term memory (Cohen, 1980). Cohen believes that the integration of such information is one of the processes of dreaming, and that the activation or increased frequency of EEG signifies a state of arousal of the brain that perhaps represents a dreaming state and a kind of reorganization or "reading" of information to be processed. The EEG features of REM, the most vivid dreaming time, include low-voltage desynchronization.

Duration and stages of sleep also vary with age even in the same individual (see Table 4.1, page 73). Mean time in bed is much higher in childhood than in adulthood, and this is not simply due to immobility. With age, the most remarkable drop in sleep duration is that of stage IV, which diminishes from an average of 115 minutes per night among persons under 5 years of age to an average of 20 minutes per night among persons 60 years of age and older (Webb and Agnew, 1971). A provocative question is whether the decline in slow wave sleep is due to diminished physical exercise among the elderly.

AGE-RELATED CHANGES IN NORMAL SLEEP

It is not just the duration of sleep that changes with age. As babies slump abruptly into quiet sleep, it is obvious that something about the character of their sleeping pattern differs from that of adults. It is not surprising that a nervous system in such a process of transition as occurs during the first year of life should certainly evolve different needs for a rest and activity cycle, and even the biological behaviors of sleep. The process of transition in the nervous system does not cease on reaching young adulthood, however. While the elderly person who falls asleep frequently during the daytime or who wanders about the house aimlessly at night may be the brunt of common jokes, it is clear that the pattern of sleeping and even the components of sleep behavior change with advanced age. The nature and time course of that evolution is not altogether clear, but certainly for the practicing physician, it is important to recognize that it exists.

The following discussion focuses predominantly on the development of normal sleep patterns in small children and then assesses some of the emerging observations about sleep in the elderly. Most of the remainder of this book deals with normal and abnormal sleep in children and adults in young or middle life, so the following may be faulted for focusing on "the beginning . . . and the end." The processes and forces giving rise to the alteration in sleep cycles is less clear, unfortunately, because to elucidate them would certainly enhance such a discussion.

Development of Normal Sleep Patterns

In rapid fashion from 24 weeks of gestation until 1 to 2 months postterm, a developing infant passes from continued presence in an atypical sleep state to a pattern of cycling between waking and two well-defined sleep states already almost completely analogous to those seen in older children and adults. Between 24 and 27 weeks' gestation, premature infants spend basically all their time in an atypical sleep state that has some features expected of early REM (active sleep) and others of non-REM (NREM, quiet sleep) (Dreyfus-Brisac, 1968). There is almost constant motor activity but only rarely does it resemble immature startles, which are sudden, brief, generalized body movements characteristic of NREM closer to term (Prechtl, Akiyama, Zinkin, et al, 1968). Rapid eye movements are rare, do not appear in bursts, and are mainly vertical. The cardiac rate is quite stable although respiration is irregular. There is no suggestion of cyclic organization and the EEG generally shows bursts of high-voltage, occipitally predominant, slow wave pleomorphic activity, alternating with long periods of very depressed activity (tracé discontinu) (Dreyfus-Brisac, 1968; Ellingson, 1975; Parmelee, Schulte, Akiyama, et al, 1968) (Figure 3.1). Chin muscle tone is almost always absent.

At about 29 weeks, REM sleep begins to emerge, characterized by increased respiratory rate, more frequent eye movements, and intermittent EEG activation. Chin muscle tone begins to appear at about 33 weeks but REM-associated drops are inconsistent until about 37 weeks (Petre-Quadens, 1967) (Figure 3.2). Respiration and heart rate are irregular and minor twitches occur randomly in different muscles. Smiling becomes associated with REM near term.

Quiet sleep, or NREM, begins to emerge as a distinct state behaviorally somewhere between 32 and 35 weeks depending on the strictness of criteria used for identification (Dreyfus-Brisac, 1970). Quiet sleep is well formed behaviorally when there is associated absence of body and eye movements (except for recurrent startles and bursts of repetitive jaw and mouth

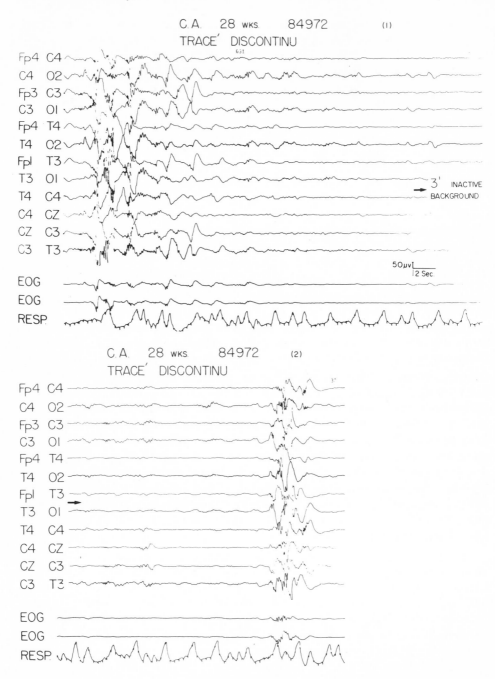

Figure 3.1. Tracé discontinu EEG pattern in a premature infant at a gestational age of 28 weeks. Two bursts of diffuse high-voltage polymorphic delta activity intermixed with faster, lower-voltage rhythmical components are seen several minutes apart on a background of markedly diminished voltage with only minimal irregular electrical activity.

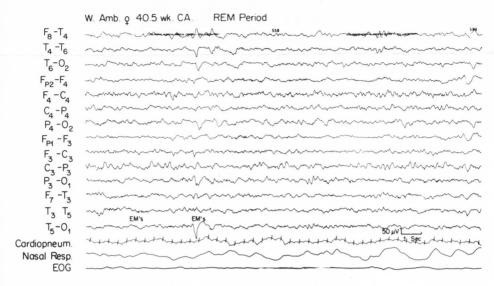

W. Amb. ♀ 40.5 wk. CA.   REM Period

F_8-T_4
T_4-T_6
T_6-O_2
$F_{P2}-F_4$
F_4-C_4
C_4-P_4
P_4-O_2
$F_{P1}-F_3$
F_3-C_3
C_3-P_3
P_3-O_1
F_7-T_3
$T_3 T_5$
T_5-O_1
Cardiopneum.
Nasal Resp.
EOG

EM's   EM's

50 µV
1 Sec

Figure 3.2. REM (active sleep) in a full-term infant. There is continuous diffuse low-voltage mixed theta and delta activity across the scalp, irregular respiration, and several eye movements. Not shown here are sections with increased eye movements, irregular heart rate, and small body movements. (Reprinted by permission of the publisher, from Lombroso, 1981.)

movements resembling, but faster than, sucking movements) (Prechtl, 1974; Wolff, 1959) with the presence of regular cardiac and respiratory patterns. An early tracé alternant EEG pattern is seen as early as 28 weeks, becomes associated with quiet sleep by 32 weeks, and appears in its mature form as 2- to 6-second bursts of high-amplitude slow waves separated by 4 to 8 seconds of low-voltage mixed activity at about 36 weeks (Parmelee et al, 1968; Dreyfus-Brisac, 1970, 1964; Lombroso, 1981) (Figure 3.3). There is now good association between behavioral and electrophysiological (EEG and electromyographical) measurements of stage (Table 3.1).

Table 3.1. Schematic Organization of the Usefulness of Measurements in Defining Sleep State in the Premature and Young Infant

	Weeks Conceptional Age					*Months Postterm*	
	24	*28*	*32*	*36*	*40*	*3*	*8*
Body movements	±	+	+ +	+ + +	+ + + +	+ + + +	+ + + +
Eye movements		+	+ +	+ + +	+ + + +	+ + + +	+ + + +
Respiration pattern			±	+ +	+ + +	+ + + +	+ + + +
EEG			±	+ +	+ + +	+ + + +	+ + + +
Chin EMG			+	+ + +	+ + + +	+ + + +	+ + + +

Reprinted by permission of the publisher, from Parmelee and Stern (1972).

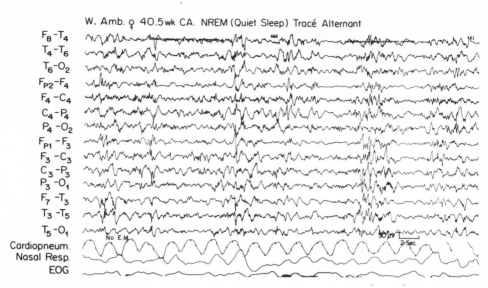

W. Amb. ♀ 40.5wk CA. NREM (Quiet Sleep) Tracé Alternant

Figure 3.3. NREM (quiet sleep) in a full-term infant. EEG shows a tracé alternant pattern with bursts of high-voltage slow waves with occasional sharper components lasting 4 to 6 seconds separated by sections with desynchronized background similar to that seen in REM. Respiration and heart rate are regular and there are no body or eye movements. (Reprinted by permission of the publisher, from Lombroso, 1981.)

Before term, most of the infant's sleep is active sleep. At 40 weeks' gestation there is a fairly equal distribution between the two sleep states. During the next 3 months, from 40 to 52 weeks, further important changes occur. Startles disappear rapidly within the first one to two weeks. At one month, sleep spindles begin to appear and are most prominent during the third and fourth months (Metcalf, 1972). Between one and two months of age, the tracé alternant pattern is replaced with a sequence of NREM stages analogous to those seen in older individuals, that is, classifiable as stages I through IV (Ellingson, 1975). At 6 months of age K-complexes first begin to appear associated with NREM sleep, and become progressively prominent until plateauing at age 2 years (Metcalf, Mondale, and Butler, 1971). Sleep cycles last about 50 minutes at term (Lenard, 1970; Stern, Parmelee, and Harris, 1973; Stern, Parmelee, Akiyama, et al, 1969), increase very slowly during the early years, and do not reach adult levels of about 90 minutes until adolescence (Williams, Karacan, and Hursch, 1974). Similarly, the percentage of sleep made up by REM slowly declines, reaching about 33 percent by age 3, 30 percent by age 5, 27 percent by age 11, and approximately adult values of 22 to 26 percent by midadolescence (Stern et al, 1969; Williams, Karacan, and Hursch, 1974; Roffwarg, Muzio, and Dement, 1966).

The full-term newborn sleeps 16 to 17 hours per day, with the sleep-wake periods being fairly evenly distributed day and night (Ellingson, 1975; Parmelee, Wenner, and Schultz, 1964). Sleep is divided into about seven episodes varying from 20 minutes to 5 or 6 hours in duration. Over the next three to four months the total number of sleep periods decreases to four or five, about two-thirds of the sleep, and the longest sleep period (up to eight or nine hours in some infants) occurs at night (Figures 3.4 and 3.5). Total sleep, however, is still about 15 hours per day (Parmelee, Wenner, and Schultz, 1964). By 3 months of age the majority of infants are already sleeping through the night at least from midnight to 5 AM (Moore and Ucko, 1957). After this age there is continued consolidation of sleep periods such that by 6 months of age a pattern is generally organized into nighttime sleep and two daytime nap periods. By 1 year of age the child is still sleeping about 14 to 15 hours a day. If the morning nap has not yet been abandoned, it most likely will be during the second year. By age 2 the child is typically sleeping 12 to 13 hours including 1 to 2 hours after lunch. Definite dream reports at this age are obtained after waking from REM (Kohler, Coddington, and Agnew, 1968). The final nap is given up at any point from age 2 to 5 years in most children, with the majority stopping at age 3 (Illingsworth, 1951).

After age 3 and until adolescence, further decreases in sleep time are slow. During latency, napping is rare and nighttime sleep gradually decreases from about 12 hours to 10 hours in the preadolescent period (Williams, Karacan, and Hursch, 1974). During the four years of puberty, rapid new changes occur. Nighttime sleep decreases further to seven or eight hours and the percentage of stage IV sleep increases, although the absolute amount of stage IV decreases (Williams, Karacan, and Hursch, 1974; Carskadon, Harvey, Duke, et al, 1980; Feinberg, 1974; Williams, Karacan, and Davis, 1972). Evidence, however, suggests this amount of sleep is culturally mediated and is inadequate (Carskadon et al, 1980; Anders, Carskadon, and Dement, 1980; Webb and Agnew, 1975). In 1910, students aged 8 to 17 averaged 1.5 hours more sleep per night than do present-day ones (Webb and Agnew, 1974). Today, adolescents are not likely to waken spontaneously on school-day mornings, and they sleep at least one hour later on the weekends (Anders, Carskadon, Dement, et al, 1978), and when given constant opportunities to sleep at night, they average about nine hours (Carskadon et al, 1980).

Sleep in the Elderly

Good information about the evolution of sleeping patterns, either normal or pathological, among the elderly is elusive. Several powerful obstacles confront the investigator of sleep disturbances in old people. These include:

1. Longitudinal studies of such behaviors as sleep would require many years, and should include control of highly variable influences such as

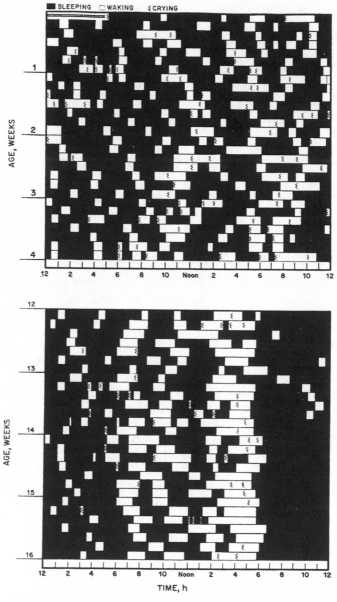

Figure 3.4.   Behavior record of one child from birth to 4 weeks and 12 to 16 weeks. Each horizontal line represents one day. Time is indicated in hours across the bottom with noon at midpoint and midnight at either end. (Reprinted by permission of the publisher from Parmelee, 1974.)

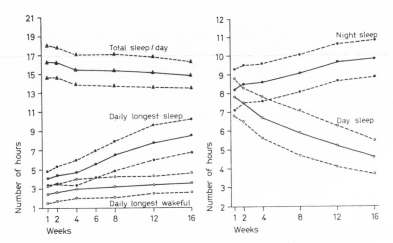

Figure 3.5. On the left, the average amount of total daily sleep from 1 to 16 weeks of age of 46 infants is illustrated in the upper half, the average daily longest sleep and wakefulness below. On the right, the average amount of sleep during the night (7 PM to 7 AM) and day (7 AM to 7 PM) from 1 to 16 weeks of age. --- = standard deviation; — = mean.) (Reprinted by permission of the publisher from Parmelee, 1974.)

diet, climate, furniture, and even economic status.

For persons now beyond the age of 60, standardized techniques and recording equipment were not even available during their younger adult years, so that the culmination of longitudinal studies must depend on initiation of such studies now.

2. Issues of informed consent clearly will bias sample selection for such a study.
3. The high incidence of chronic illness or subtle deterioration in any of a number of organ systems not recognized at entrance to a study casts doubt on the possibility of a true control group among elderly people.

The following problems also complicate the interpretation of sleep patterns in the elderly:

1. How does the investigator distinguish the effects of disease from the effects of maturation in the aged?
2. Relevant pathology of sleep may not cause symptoms, and so from the individual's comfort or reports, it may be difficult to tell normal from pathological sleep.
3. As Howard points out in Chapter 9, sleep recordings in the sleep laboratory are very expensive and labor-intensive, and they are carried out in surroundings not familiar to the individual and therefore raise

the question of introducing slight changes in the person's sleeping patterns. Furthermore, such laboratory recordings are usually less than 24-hour cycles. Circadian rhythm functions may be particularly relevant among the aged, and yet 24-hour recording practices are only emerging at the present.

It is clear that old people complain more about their sleep than do younger persons. As early as 1931, Laird noted that sleep latency and wakings after sleep onset (WASO) increased in older men. It is clear from literally hundreds of studies of the subjective assessments in the elderly that satisfaction with sleep is generally very low in this population (Miles and Dement, 1980). It is still difficult, if not impossible, to distinguish whether indeed the biological need for sleep simply diminishes with age, or whether the processes of aging (or exposure to disease among the aged population) interfere with sleep. That is, does the older person, accustomed to the sleeping habits of younger years, complain because sleep habits have become different, or because they have become pathological. Stated otherwise, it is unclear, "whether the sleep of the elderly is pathological or merely different" (Miles and Dement, 1980).

Changes in Sleep Patterns of Age

While it seems universally agreed that the time spent in bed is greater among the elderly (see Table 4.1, page 000) the efficiency index of sleep is lower so that the sleep period time (SPT) diminishes (Miles and Dement, 1980; Williams, Karacan, and Hursch, 1970). Beyond the age of 65 years sleep latency increases, the WASO increases, and the duration of time while still in bed but after awakening in the morning also increases.

The most striking interruption of sleep in the elderly seems to be with the number and duration of wakings after onset of sleep, the WASO. Since most sleep laboratories require at least 30 seconds in order to score a change in sleep stage, brief awakenings, 29 seconds or less, will often be omitted, so that conventional means of scoring brief wakings are, if anything, conservative. Prinz, Peskin, Vitaliano, et al (1982) reported an average of 6.8 arousals in elderly subjects, with a mean duration of more than 7 minutes.

Although the frequency and voltage of EEG background activity decrease in both sleep and wakefulness, the voltage and duration of slow wave sleep are significantly reduced in older patients. Kales et al (1967) found that the percentage of stage III sleep was similar to that of young adults, but stage IV consisted of only 1.4 percent of total sleep time compared to 11 percent for younger subjects. Others have found similar reductions in total stage IV sleep (Feinberg, 1974; Kales et al, 1967; Kahn and Fisher, 1969; Kahn, Fisher, and Lieberman, 1970).

Whereas REM sleep undergoes considerable change during age in cats and rodents, such changes are less clear in elderly humans. Although the number of REM periods drops from about seven in small children to about four or five periods in older children, it stays constant throughout the remainder of life. The average length of REM period drops significantly in some individuals, but may not drop enough in the elderly to be certain that this truly represents a change in sleep stage characteristics.

Miles and Dement (1980) reviewed other physiological functions that change during sleep in the elderly. Foremost among these are respiration and especially the number of hypopneas. The higher incidence of respiratory diseases as well as respiratory pauses raises the cogent and obviously important question of the role of respiratory deterioration as the cause of any definable deterioration in sleeping rather than a primary evolution in respiratory patterns per se.

Relationship Between Daytime Napping and Nocturnal Sleep

If elderly people, especially those who complain of poor nocturnal sleep, are studied, the incidence, and indeed intrusion, of brief sleeping episodes during the day is quite prevalent. These have been called "microsleeps" and can be defined not only by momentary inattentiveness, but by electrographic evidence of stage II and even occasionally REM sleep. Although these daytime microsleeps seem to occur less often in persons given sedatives to deepen sleep during the night, they continue to some degree. It is difficult to determine whether these episodes result from partial sleep deprivation due to poorly sustained nocturnal sleep, or whether they diminish the nocturnal drive for sleep among the elderly.

Miles and Dement proffer several theories regarding the observed changes in polygraphically recorded sleep among the elderly:

1. The need or drive for slow wave sleep and long periods of uninterrupted sleep change or diminish in senescence.
2. The requirements for slow wave sleep or prolonged uninterrupted periods of sleep still continue as they do at younger ages, but for some reason are not fulfilled. That is, sleep remains necessary and in some manner restorative, but cannot satisfactorily be maintained in the elderly because of underlying or coexistent physical or mental disease, age-determined deterioration, or loss of circadian regulation from age.
3. The requirement or drive for sleep both in duration and type is different among the elderly than among younger people. Miles and Dement see the possibility that old people in more primitive societies needed to sleep more lightly because they could not escape danger as rapidly when it approached, so that they needed a head start on arousal. Such a characteristic might be an evolutionary or survival advantage

to any society that relied heavily on its aged members, say for advice or wise counsel.

4. The need for sleep continues as in younger ages, and is in fact, being fulfilled, but measurements applied arbitrarily in our laboratories do not reflect the process as accurately for older people as for younger ones. This argument is probably not very persuasive, since the elderly in fact complain about changes in sleep.

5. Naps during the day, frequent microsleeps, sedentary behavior, and psychosocial factors affect the nocturnal sleep of the aged more than they do young people. Forced inactivity, retirement, and social expectations of the "sleepy grandfather" would all seem to contribute to this possible explanation.

As mentioned throughout this book, it is important to recognize that sleep is merely one aspect of a total circadian cycle. If changes in sleep actually occur among the aged, and they seem to in humans, then areas requiring exploration include deterioration of a 24-hour or even annual internal pacemaker; a change or alteration in the frequency of the pacemaker that would predispose to dissociation of certain rhythms; a diminished general level of sensory-specific responses rendering an older person less affected by zeitgebers; and changes in the environment that deprive elderly persons of normally effective zeitgebers.

Much remains to be learned about changes in time and activity needs of the elderly; however, many methodological problems stand in the way of making such studies. Nonetheless, it is obvious that sleep-wake function and especially satisfaction with nocturnal sleep are among the most important concerns for which elderly persons seek medical advice. Unfortunately, medications that influence sleep often have particularly hazardous influences on the elderly, and are too readily supplied by physicians and accepted by the patient. Recognizing the changes of sleep patterns that occur with age reinforces the concept that sleep is an energy-consuming process that is reactive to the life environment. The physician caring for a person with complaints of sleep needs to be aware not only of the influence of daytime environment, but the age of the patient and the relevance of this complaint to the person's overall level of function.

BIOLOGICAL STAGES OF SLEEP

Although they are helpful in identifying physiological phases of sleep, electrical recording devices may have in part diverted attention from certain important characteristics of sleep by focusing more on recordable epiphenomena than on body movements, endocrine functions, or total organism behavior. In other words, the conventional methods of determining sleep staging may be misleading for a biological understanding of sleep (Parmeggiani, 1980). Types and intensity of body motion certainly pertain to the degree of activation, or physiological state of the person, and may be more relevant to what people recognize as satisfactory or restful sleep than are such observations as EEG tracings. Hobson, Spagna, and Malenka (1978), for example, showed that there were phases of immobility alternating intermittently with varying types and degrees of movement throughout the night. There was a correlation between phases of movement or immobility and the stages of sleep as defined by conventional polygraphic recording, but there were times that body movement or immobility could not be predicted adequately by sleep stages. Periods of immobility of 30 minutes or longer occurred intermittently throughout the night and were more associated with slow wave sleep or descending stage II than with any other phases. Most especially, body movement, particularly of a phasic or repetitive rapid type, occurred most often during REM sleep. The subjective assessment of satisfaction or "goodness" of sleep was higher if the individual awakened from a phase of immobility or after a night with many long immobility phases. These studies showed not only that there was some correlation between body movement and activity and the conventionally defined phases of sleep, but that the degree of body mobility was more important for satisfaction of sleep than the phases defined polygraphically.

The number of sleep stage changes is influenced not only by the ambient noise and activity level in the laboratory, but by the degree of anxiety, agitation, and activity level experienced by individual during the preceding day (Webb and Agnew, 1971). The amount of physical exercise during a waking interval certainly influences the quality of sleep as well, perhaps more than emotional stress. Sleep latency is briefer and total sleep time is increased in response to physical exercise, and the slow wave sleep fraction is especially increased after exercise (Hobson, 1968; Matsumoto, Nishiho, Suto, et al, 1968; Baekeland and Lasky, 1968). Sleep latency is usually briefer immediately after sexual activity, and in the rat it appears that the proportion of slow wave sleep increases after sexual activity (Boland and Dewsbury, 1971). This may explain a common tendency to fall asleep after coitus.

Dietary influences certainly influence sleep behavior. Hartmann has suggested that the amino acid L-tryptophan, as a precursor of 5-hydroxytryptamine, may induce sleep by increasing the available amount of an important neurotransmitter (Hartmann, Cravens, and List, 1974; Hartmann and Elion, 1977). Administering purified tryptamine or tryptophan or foods rich in these amino acids has provided somewhat erratic results, however. The sheer influence of starvation also seems to increase not only the duration of sleep, but the percentage of slow wave sleep (Oswald, 1972). If slow wave sleep spares protein, Oswald argues that this form of sleep may be protective in the starving animal.

Sleep Responsiveness

The duration of sleep and the time required to fall asleep are influenced by the preceding waking interval. Total sleep time and the amount of slow wave sleep are proportional to the duration of wakefulness before sleep. Sleep latency is shorter following longer periods of wakefulness or sleep deprivation (Mendelson, Gillin, and Wyatt, 1977). It is not simply the duration of wakefulness or sleep deprivation that is pertinent, however; clearly, the time of day that sleep is attempted is critical. Sleep latency is much shorter at night than in the daytime. In equally darkened rooms, a person accustomed to sleeping at night, even after prolonged sleep deprivation, falls asleep more rapidly during nocturnal hours than during daytime hours. In contrast to slow wave sleep, total sleep time, and latency of sleep onset, the duration and latency of onset of REM sleep seem not to be significantly influenced by the amount of daytime activity or physical exercise, or usually by the amount of emotional stress. Rather, REM sleep seems more entrained or influenced by a 24-hour rhythm or circadian effect. Naps taken in the morning have more numerous REM periods and more total REM time than naps taken in the afternoon; and neither has as much REM as nighttime sleep (Mendelson, Gillin, Wyatt, 1977; Karacan, Williams, Finley, et al, 1970).

Sleep Deprivation in Normal Subjects

Much of the information and speculation about various sleep phases and physiological sleep functions are based on studies of sleep deprivation. For many reasons, behaviors and sleep records of people deprived of sleep may be misleading or not be truly relevant to normal physiology of sleep. For example, sleep deprivation alone causes a lower-voltage and less persistent alpha rhythm in the EEG, even while the subject is awake, without any changes in the level of alertness. Superficial review of an EEG of a person with diminished alpha rhythm may be misinterpreted as the onset of stage I sleep.

Aside from total sleep deprivation, selective deprivation of REM sleep has drawn the greatest amount of attention. Earliest studies suggested that REM deprivation causes more or less specific psychological aberrations, predominantly irritability, inability to concentrate, hallucinations, and nervousness (Sampson, 1965). Because of hallucinations and lack of concentration, the traits seen after REM deprivation were interpreted as a disturbance of thought process. It was concluded that one function of REM sleep was a kind of integration process, the coupling of thought and affect, which is necessary for normal function while awake. In fact, the REM deprivation model initially received some enthusiastic support as a model for schizophrenia. Subsequent studies, however, have not shown such uniform changes with selective REM deprivation if total sleep time is maintained in the normal range (Kales, Hoedemaker, and Jacobson, 1964; Foulkes, Pivik, and Ahrens, 1968). It now seems unlikely that REM sleep deprivation, at least in intermittent or isolated intrusions, produces serious or lasting psychological problems (Mendelson, Gillin, and Wyatt, 1977). Even the theory of total sleep deprivation as a presumed cause of psychosis (Dement, 1960) has basically fallen by the wayside. Other than irritability, daydreaming, and isolated hallucinatory experiences, true psychiatric disorders have not been found to result from sleep deprivation in humans. A recent study by Rechtschaffen (1983), however, does suggest total sleep deprivation may in fact be dangerous for mammals (see Chapter 1). Although hallucinations are not to be denied, especially among shift workers or people who work longer than 24 hours at a time, these often can be shown to represent "mini-sleep" experiences. They are almost always discerned by the individual as being related to a severely drowsy period. They are distinguished from pathological hallucinations by being immediately recognized by the subject as imaginary events.

Certainly, it is not to be denied that chronic sleep deprivation may lead to depression or continuous irritability, but it does not lead to actual psychosis. Of 350 people totally deprived of sleep for 112 hours, only 7 had evidence of psychotic behavior (Tyler, 1958), and there was no control for thought disorders among subjects prior to the experiment. Even violent outbursts were at times included among psychotic behaviors. It is conceivable that some of these may have simply represented excessive irritability.

Selective REM deprivation does suggest increased cortical excitability in animal studies (Owen and Bliss, 1970), and it seems to increase stimulus-induced aggressive behaviors, which may be manifested as short temper, impulsivity, or suspiciousness (Morden, Connor, Mitchell, et al, 1968). Sexual behavior or sexual craving seems to be increased after selective REM deprivation (Dement, 1965). Most studies in this area have methodological problems, which include some interruption of other sleep phases, forcing the subject to sleep in an artificial environment, restriction upon mobility, or occasionally rather imprecise definitions of REM sleep. It is clear, however, that selective REM deprivation does in some manner interfere with behavior, affect, and processing of information and emotion. With this in mind, it is obvious that a regulatory process is required to balance the several qualitatively different sleep phases. Whenever a person is deprived of a particular stage of sleep, an excess or compensatory amount of that stage will occur when uninhibited sleep is permitted thereafter. In other words, when a person selectively deprived of stage II sleep for several nights is left to sleep uninterruptedly, there will be an increase in the amount of stage II sleep, perhaps causing either a longer duration of total sleep or an increase of the depleted stage at the expense of other stages, most often stage I or REM. This rebound phenomenon is more visible with slow wave or REM sleep than with other stages.

Perhaps because of the association of REM sleep with dreaming and concern in this century with dreams, a focus on rebound properties after REM sleep deprivation has led to an interest in a property called REM pressure. When deprived of REM sleep for several nights, not only will a person have a rebound increase in the amount of REM sleep on subsequent nights, but it will take progressively stronger or more numerous stimuli to continue to deprive that individual of REM sleep. That is, once there is a deficit of REM sleep, it becomes harder and harder to prevent its emergence. The concept of REM pressure is that there is an underlying force from the central nervous system to generate more REM. When unleashed, this pressure gives rise not only to a rebound in the duration of REM sleep, but to some kind of vigor or intensity of the state.

This is exemplified by the rebound of REM sleep when a suppressant is stopped. When medication such as a tricyclic antidepressant compound or alcohol is initiated, the onset and duration of REM sleep are suppressed. As the suppressant is continued, the REM pressure gradually forces the pattern back to the normal amount of REM sleep for that individual. When the suppressant is discontinued, the increased physiological pressure to restore REM sleep leads to a rebound effect, experienced as longer and more intense REM sleep and causing nightmares and unpleasant sleep.

Zeitgebers

Since sleep is a reactive behavior, its intrinsic regulators must be modulated by external time markers called *zeitgebers*. These are signs of diurnal sequence, such as sunset, rooster crowing, subway rumbling, and the like. The zeitgebers' influences are also mediated by endocrine or metabolic responses to general environment or climate. For example, during the cold, inhospitable winter season, with longer nights, shorter hunting hours in the daylight, and presumably a diminished food supply, it is to daylight animals' (and humans') advantage to sleep longer. Accordingly, during warmer seasons with longer days, sleep should be affected in a manner that allows for more harvesting and perhaps storage of food. Outside time clues are particularly influential on those phases of the cycle preparing for sleep and for awakening. Light seems to be the most effective pacesetter for sleep, probably because it is the most reliable predictor not only of day but also of seasonal and (hence survival) changes.

For humans, however, socially pertinent zeitgebers are infinitely more effective for entrainment of the sleeping phases in the sleep-wake cycle. Such clues as audible street traffic sounds, voices of people in adjacent rooms, radio or television broadcasts, and aromas signifying presence of food or beverage are much more effective for engendering sleepiness or for terminating a sleep cycle than are changes in light and dark or pure sounds. Wever (1979) showed that a sound made by a metal gong was perceived as a social type of signal and was much more effective for altering sleeping-waking behavior than was a pure tone of even much higher intensity. Even

12-hour shifts in dark-light or sleep-wake cycles are accommodated within four to six days in transcontinental travelers (the condition called jet lag) who go from one social context to another, whereas such schedule shifts often require much longer periods of adjustment when performed in laboratory or isolation circumstances. In the laboratory the zeitgebers are less social even if more discrete.

Temporal Isolation and Free-running Cycles

From a different perspective than that of deprivation studies, isolation of the person or organism from outside time clues tells a good deal about the intrinsic regulatory mechanisms of sleep. Weitzman (1981) says that temporal isolation sleep studies that show an intrinsic maintenance mechanism to sleep phases and timed regulation demonstrate that there is a logic and most especially a regulator of sleep-wake cycles. Hence the sleep process can be called a "lawful" biological function that fulfills certain measurable physical, biochemical, and behavioral principles, just as free bodies in space follow certain laws of physics that dictate their responses. Aschoff (1969) and Weber and associates (1980) were the first to show that human sleep-wake cycles last significantly longer than 24 hours if allowed so-called free running. That is, if zeitgebers symbolizing outside time are eliminated, human cycles last consistently longer than 24 hours. Other studies have been confirmatory.

The initial isolation studies were performed in caves that usually were cold and uncomfortable; subjects slept and conducted their activities in tents. More recent studies have been performed in elaborate laboratory units that are a good deal more comfortable and include indoor plumbing, piped-in music, and even television for recreation. Clearly such different settings provide for different atmospheres, and yet the results from isolation studies in either environment have shown cycles lasting longer than 24 hours, which are called hypernychthemeral.

In an early subject isolated from outside time clues for five months, the average circadian period was 27.2 hours. Wever (1979) reported a subject in a time-isolation environment whose cycle was entrained to 24 hours by a fixed signal. He was perfectly comfortable as the zeitgeber was progressively slowed to 24.6 hours without his knowledge, and he did not report being aware of the change. Having become acclimated to the 24.6-hour cycle, the subject reported feeling irritable and morose when the zeitgeber without his knowledge was changed back to 24 hours. Weber et al (1980) reported two people who had hypernychthemeral cycles despite living in environments with normal light-dark and social cues. One subject had maintained such a cycle for more than four years and yet had been able to keep up with social contacts and work. Both subjects could force themselves to perform under 24-hour cycles when required, but were less comfortable and felt less productive than when allowed to set their own longer sleeping and

waking times. One of these subjects, a male student who was studied between ages 24 and 28 years, had an average sleep-wake cycle of 26.5 hours
and an average sleep time of 7.6 hours per day, although his range was from
6 to 8.6 hours of sleep per day.

In another study, ten healthy adults stayed in temporal isolation in
comfortable living quarters for periods between 15 and 105 days (Wever,
1979). There was a good deal of variation among them, but the average
circadian cycle was 25 hours, with few subjects having a cycle less than 24
hours. Initially, subjects maintained sleep-wake cycles very nearly at 24
hours, paralleling their normal day-night schedule. After variable periods
of free running (isolation from zeitgebers), most developed cycles of long
biological days, often greater than 35 hours, which sometimes alternated
with shorter days of 25 hours or less. Within the free-running times, although the ratio of sleep to total time remained constant, the onset of the
sleep periods seemed to occur at a specific phase or phase angle of an
internal circadian rhythm, which was paralleled by body temperature. Although very long biological days included much longer sleep periods than
short biological days, the onset of sleep with both seemed to occur 180
degrees out of phase of the temperature cycle, so that a steady length of
time between the sleep phases was maintained. In a free-running environment, REM sleep seemed to occur earlier in the sleep period, being more
prominent in the first three hours than in a conventional, controlled sleep
environment. Under free running, at a particular phase in temperature
change, REM sleep could be predicted for each individual. Slow wave sleep,
by contrast, was not dependent on a particular sleep onset phase, but more
on total elapsed time from the previous phase. This effect of time cycles
upon REM and slow wave sleep was interpreted to mean that REM was
somehow related to an overall biological signal, whereas slow wave sleep
was more dependent upon current activity and prior effects of sleep.

Core body temperature seemed to have a 24-hour rhythm irrespective
of sleeping and waking cycles. Some measurable endocrine functions resembled REM sleep as independent biological rhythms, whereas others seemed
tied to specific sleep phases, differing from one free-running day to the next
depending on the sleep cycle. Levels of serum cortisol, for example, had a
six- to eight-hour peak preceding onset of sleep, and another peak, lower
in intensity, at onset of sleep. Serum cortisol secretion followed a cycle
similar to that of body temperature. Growth hormone, by contrast, continued its major secretory peak two hours after the onset of slow wave sleep
whenever this occurred, whether in long or short biological days.

In view of the varying responses of sleep phases during free running,
Czeisler et al (1980) showed that REM and other circadian rhythms usually
cluster not only around a circadian cycle, but are coupled in response to
environmental cues. In the free-running time-isolated environment, REM
and these other functions became uncoupled because the time clues that
held them together were removed (Kronauer, Czeisler, Pilatos, et al, 1982).

Even with constant bedrest and virtually no somatic activity, body temperature has a diurnal cycle. More than 100 physiological variables have been shown to be rhythmical over a 24-hour period, most of which have cycles longer than 24 hours if time clues are removed. Wever (1979) argues that even readiness for single events such as birth or death follow proscribed daily rhythms. While a high degree of phase constancy is necessary for survival, nonetheless, there must be some adaptability to survive in changing environments. For example, the constant body temperature cycle may be influenced significantly by ingestion of food, and entrainment of the diurnal cycle may be compressed by dependence on light. It is probably biologically advantageous to have a recurrent oscillating cycle longer than the environmental cycle that can be compressed by outside clues.

In a formula advanced by Pittendrigh (1979), *tau* as the period of sleep-wake cycle is proportional to a delay-advance relationship, such that tau is a constant depending upon delay-advance flexibility. Light as influence can only shorten tau when the delay-advance constant is very short. In nocturnal organisms, increased or constant light lengthens tau, whereas in diurnal animals increased light shortens tau. Thus light as a zeitgeber or time regulator would be particularly important and effective for compressing a sleep period. If there were a drive, for example, to a 26-hour, hypernychthemeral cycle, a diminished duration of light stimulus would allow the prolonged cycle and accompanying longer duration of sleep, but as days grow longer into summer season, the cycle, particularly the sleeping phase, would be adjustable. The effect of environment on overt biological rhythms may not be simple or direct, but the environment affects other biological oscillators, which in turn have effects on one another and on eventual overt biological rhythms.

REFERENCES

Anders TF, Carskadon MA, Dement WC. Sleep and sleepiness in children and adolescents. Pediatr Clin North Am 1980;27(1):29–43.

Anders TF, Carskadon MA, Dement WC, Harvey K. Sleep habits of children and the identification of pathologically sleepy children. Child Psychiatry Hum Dev 1978;9:56–63.

Aschoff J. Desynchronization and resynchronization of human circadian rhythms. Aerospace Med 1969;40:844–49.

Baekeland F, Lasky R. Exercise and sleep patterns in college athletes. Percept Motor Skills 1968;23:1203–7.

Boland B, Dewsbury D. Characteristics of sleep following sexual activity and wheel running in male rats. Physiol Behav 1971;6:145–49.

Carskadon MA, Harvey K, Duke P, Anders TF, Latt IF, Dement WC. Pubertal changes in daytime sleepiness. Sleep 1980;2(4):453–60.

Cohen DB. The cognitive activity of sleep. Prog Brain Res 1980;53:307–24.

Czeisler CA, Zimmerman J, Ronda J, Moore-Ede M, Weitzman ED. Timing of

REM sleep coupled to the circadian rhythm of body temperature in man. Sleep 1980;2:329–56.

Dement WC.The effect of dream deprivation. Science 1960;131:1705–8.

Dement WC. Recent studies on the biological role of rapid eye movement sleep. Am J Psychiatry 1965;122:404–8.

Dreyfus-Brisac C. The electroencephalogram of the premature infant and the full-term newborn. In: Kellaway P, Petersen I, eds. Neurologic and electroencephalographic correlative studies in infancy. New York: Grune & Stratton, 1964:186.

Dreyfus-Brisac C. Sleep ontogenesis in early human prematurity from 24–27 weeks of conceptual age. Dev Psychobiol 1968;2(3):162–69.

Dreyfus-Brisac C. Ontogenesis of sleep in human prematures after 32 weeks of conceptual age. Dev Psychobiol 1970;3(2):91–121.

Ellingson RJ. Ontogenesis of sleep in the human. In: Lairy GC, Salzarulo P, eds. Experimental study of human sleep: methodical problems. Amsterdam: Elsevier, 1975:120–40.

Feinberg I. Changes in sleep cycle patterns with age. J Psychiatr Res 1974;10:272–306.

Foulkes D, Pivik T, Ahrens J. Effects of "dream deprivation" on dream content; an attempted cross-night replication. J Abnorm Psychiatry 1968;73:403–15.

Hartmann E, Baekeland F, Zwilling G. Psychological differences between long and short sleepers. Arch Gen Psychiatry 1972;26:463–68.

Hartmann E, Cravens J, List S. Hypnotic effects of L-tryptophan. Arch Gen Psychiatry 1974;31:394–97.

Hartmann E, Elion R. The insomnia of "sleeping in a strange place"; effects on L-tryptophan. Psychopharmacology 1977;53:131–33.

Hobson JA. Sleep after exercise. Science 1968;162:1503–5.

Hobson JA, Spagna T, Malenka R. Ethology of sleep studied with time-lapse photography: postural immobility and sleep-cycle phase in humans. Science 1978;201:1251–53.

Illingsworth RS. Sleep problems in the first three years. Br Med J 1951;1:722–28.

Kahn E, Fisher C. The sleep characteristics of the normal aged male. J Nerv Ment Dis 1969;148:474–94.

Kahn E, Fisher C. Lieberman L. Sleep characteristics of the human aged female. Compr Psychiatry 1970;11:274–78.

Kales A, Hoedemaker F, Jacobson A. Dream deprivation: an experimental reappraisal. Nature 1964;204:1337–38.

Kales A, Wilson T, Kales J, et al. Measurements of all-night sleep on normal elderly persons. Effects of aging. J Am Geriatr Soc 1967;15:405–14.

Karacan I, Williams R, Finley W, Hursch CJ. The effects of naps on nocturnal sleep. Biol Psychiatry 1970;2:381–99.

Kohler WC, Coddington D, Agnew HW. Sleep patterns in 2-year-old children. J Pediatr 1968;72:228–33.

Kronauer R, Czeisler C, Pilatos S, Moore-Ede M, Weitzman E. Mathematical model of the human circadian system with two interacting oscillators. Am J Physiol 1982;242:R3–17.

Laird D. A survey of the sleep habits of 509 men of distinction. Am J Med 1931;26:271–74.

Lenard HG. Sleep studies in infancy. Acta Paediatr Scand 1970;59:572–81.

Lombroso CT. Normal and abnormal EEGs in full-term neonates. In: Henry C, ed. Current clinical neurophysiology. Amsterdam: Elsevier, 1981:83–150.

Matsumoto J, Nishiho T, Suto T, Sadahiro T, Miyoshi M. Influence of fatigue on sleep. Nature 1968;218:177–78.

Meddis R, Pearson A, Langford G. An extreme case of healthy insomnia. Electroencephalogr Clin Neurophysiol 1973;35:213–14.

Mendelson W, Gillin J, Wyatt R. Human sleep and its disorders. New York: Plenum Press, 1977.

Metcalf D. Sleep spindle ontogenesis in normal children. In: Smith W, ed. Drugs, development, and cerebral function. Springfield, Ill.: Charles C Thomas, 1972:125–44.

Metcalf D, Mondale J, Butler F. Ontogenesis of spontaneous K-complexes. Psychophysiology 1971;8:340–47.

Miles LE, Dement WC. Sleep and aging. Sleep 1980;101:911–17.

Moore T, Ucko LE. Nightwaking in early infancy. Part 1. Arch Dis Child 1957;32:333–42.

Morden B, Conner R, Mitchell G, Dement WC. Effects of rapid eye movement (REM) sleep deprivation on shock-induced fighting. Physiol Behav 1968;3:425–32.

Oswald I. Report to the first European congress of sleep research, Basel, Switzerland, October 3–6, 1972. Basel: S. Karger, 1973.

Owen M, Bliss EL. Sleep loss and cerebral excitability. Am J Physiol 1970;218:171–73.

Parmeggiani P. Behavioral phenomenology of sleep (somatic and vegetative). Experientia 1980;36:6–11.

Parmelee AH. Ontogeny of sleep patterns and associated periodicity in infants. In: Falkner F, Kretchmer N, Rossi E, eds. Pre- and postnatal development of the human brain. Basel: S. Karger, 1974:298–311.

Parmelee AH, Schulte FJ, Akiyama Y, Wenner WH, Schultz MA, Stern E. Maturation of EEG activity during sleep in premature infants. Electroencephalogr Clin Neurophysiol 1968;24:319–29.

Parmelee AH, Stern B. Development of states in infants. In: Clemente C, Purpura D, Mayer F, eds. Sleep and the maturing nervous system. New York: Academic Press, 1972:199–215.

Parmelee AH, Wenner WH, Schultz HR. Infant sleep patterns: from birth to 16 weeks. J Pediatr 1964;65(4):576–82.

Petre-Quadens O. Ontogenesis of paradoxical sleep in the human newborn. J Neurol Sci 1967;4:151–53.

Pittendrigh CS. Some functional aspects of circadian pacemakers. In: Suda M, Hayaishi O, Nakagawa H, eds. Biological rhythms and their central mechanisms. Amsterdam: Elsevier, 1979:3–15.

Prechtl HFR. The behavioral states of the newborn (a review). Brain Res 1974;76:185–212.

Prechtl HFR, Akiyama Y, Zinkin P, Grant DK. Polygraphic studies of the full-term newborn. I. Technical aspects of qualitative analysis. In: MacKeith R, Bax M, eds. Studies in infancy (Spastics International Medical Publications) Clin Med 1968;27:1–21.

Prinz PN, Peskin ER, Vitaliano PP, Raskind MA, Eisdorfer C. Changes in the sleep and waking EEGs in elderly subjects. J Am Geriatr Soc 1981;30:86–93.

Ragins N, Schachter S. A study of sleep behavior in two-year-old children. J Am Acad Child Psychiatry 1971;10:464–80.

Rechtschaffen A, Gilliland MA, Bergmann BM, Winter JB. Physiological correlates of prolonged sleep deprivation in rats. Science 1983;221:182–4.

Roffwarg HP, Muzio JN, Dement WC. Ontogenetic development of the human sleep-dream cycle. Science 1966;152:603–19.

Sampson H. Deprivation of dreaming sleep by two methods. I. Compensatory REM time. Arch Gen Psychiatry 1965;13:79–86.

Shepherd F. Disturbed sleep in infancy and childhood. Hatfield, England:1948.

Stern E, Parmelee AH, Akiyama Y, Schultz MA, Wenner WH. Sleep cycle characteristics in infants. Pediatrics 1969;43:65–70.

Stern E, Parmelee AH, Harris MA. Sleep state periodicity in prematures and young infants. Dev Psychobiol 1973;6(4):357–65.

Tyler DB. Psychological changes during experimental sleep deprivation. Dis Nerv Syst 1958;16:293–99.

Valatx JL, Bugat R. Genetic factors as determinants of the waking-sleeping cycle in the mouse. Brain Res 1974;69:315–50.

Webb WB, Agnew HW. Stage for sleep: influence of time course variables. Science 1971;174:1354–56.

Webb W, Agnew HW. Are we chronically sleep deprived? Bull Psychosom Soc 1975;6:47–48.

Weber AL, Cary MS, Connor N, Keyes P. Human non-24-hour sleep-wake cycles in everyday environment. Sleep 1980;2:347–54.

Weitzman ED. Sleep and its disorders. Annu Rev Neurosci 1981;4:381–417.

Wever RA. The circadian system of man: results of experiments under temporal isolation. New York: Springer-Verlag, 1979.

Williams RL, Karacan I, Davis G. Sleep patterns of pubertal males. Pediatr Res 1972;6:643–47.

Williams RL, Karacan I, Hursch CJ. Electroencephalography of human sleep; clinical applications. New York: John Wiley & Sons, 1970.

Williams RL, Karacan I, Hursch CJ. Electroencephalography of human sleep: clinical applications. New York: John Wiley & Sons, 1974.

Wolff PH. Observations on newborn infants. Psychosom Med 1959;21:110–18.

CHAPTER 4

Normal Sleep Patterns
Terrence L. Riley

In comfortable normal sleep, humans past infancy go through a sequence beginning with a period of lowered vigilance or gradual blurring of consciousness (drowsiness) followed by actual loss of consciousness after about eight minutes. The normal individual at night remains in bed for six to ten hours, awakening briefly two or three times during the night, and coming to full wakefulness spontaneously or in response to a zeitgeber (time cue) such as daylight, an alarm clock, or baby's crying. Careful observation of photographs shows that people readjust position in bed and shuffle in posture for 15 to 30 minutes, pass through an epoch of total immobility for an interval of 10 to 30 minutes, again become restive, and then gradually become totally limp in body tone. Paradoxically, during the most limp stage, humans and other mammals have rapid body twitches, moaning, movements of the eyes under the lids, and evidence of autonomic or psychic activation. Autonomic evidence may consist of penile erection, piloerection, increased heart rate, perspiration, or changes in blood pressure. The twitching of the eyes and grimacing facial expressions occur in 1- to 6-second clusters at 20- to 60-second intervals and may appear to suggest emotional activation during this particular phase of sleep, which has come to be known as rapid eye movement (REM) sleep or paradoxical sleep in animals. On awakening spontaneously or being awakened during this active phase of sleep, the subject may remark about a vivid or coherent dream. The cycle of different levels of activity is more evident in some persons than in others, and occasionally is not visible by simply watching the individual or recording movement in bed. When visible, however, the cycles last between 60 and 90 minutes and may occur three to five times during a typical night's sleep. The periods of immobility are somewhat longer and more notable during the first half of the night, and the periods of paradoxically increased activity or REM sleep are longer, the facial grimaces and eye movements more intense, later in the night.

As Loomis, Harvey, and Hobart noted in 1937, characteristic electroencephalographic (EEG) patterns accompany each of the sleep stages, even in an individual who remains basically immobile throughout the entire night. Even without changes in posture, the systematic sequence of different physiological states or EEG stages proceeds. To be sure, the frequency spectrum of brain waves varies from person to person, and the normal sequence of sleep patterns changes throughout life. Nonetheless, distinguishable, definable stages of physiological activity persist at all ages.

Although EEG characteristics are the primary criteria for defining sleep stages, they are not adequate alone to define sleep. Transitions between stages as defined by EEG often are not abrupt and may be unclear, and in fact, other body functions are frequently more important markers. By recording eye movements with cutaneous periorbital electrodes and recording neck or face muscles with transcutaneous electromyographic (EMG) recording electrodes, the reliability of polygraphic recording is increased (Dement and Kleitman, 1957). Gradual evolution of the criteria devised by Dement and Kleitman eventually led to a standardized technique published by a committee of investigators working under the auspices of the National Institutes of Neurological Diseases and Blindness (NINDB) in 1968, *A Manual of Standardized Terminology, Techniques and the Scoring System for Sleep Stages of Human Subjects* (Rechtschaffen and Kales, 1968). This still remains the basic guideline for sleep staging.

The classification described here is fundamentally based upon the manual techniques suggested by Williams, Karacan, and Hursch (1974) and Guilleminault (1982). The recording method usually used requires a polygraph with conventional EEG channels, typically with alternating-current (AC)-coupled amplifiers, and often some additional channels with direct-current (DC)-coupled amplifiers. The latter amplifiers may be necessary to record very slowly changing potentials, such as galvanic skin response and breathing rates. Inasmuch as other records are often as important as the EEG in defining sleep stage, the somewhat stilted word polysomnogram is usually used instead of terms such as all-night EEG.

The approach generally followed for staging sleep is epoch by epoch, recommended by Rechtschaffen and Kales (1968). Since brain waves are variable and discontinuous, significant staging usually is done for epochs of 30 to 60 seconds, the time filling one page or 30 cm of recording paper in commonly used polygraph instruments, or EEG machines. In addition to the stages described, one called indeterminate or movement time (MT) is often used for intervals that produce so much EEG artifact from movement that cerebral state cannot be determined. Such epochs occur particularly in the early hours of sleep or at transition times. Since the patient does not always become conscious or alert at electrographical awakening, so such MT intervals must be distinguished from movement arousals or from mere individual body movements that may be of quite short duration. For example, MT intervals may last two or three minutes.

CHARACTERISTICS OF THE BASIC
SLEEP-WAKE CYCLE

Stage 0 or W (Wakefulness)

The EEG of the waking adult or child is characterized by a generally low-voltage pattern, with scalp voltages seldom exceeding 70 μV and frequencies ranging between 4 and 25 cycles per second, or Hertz (Hz). Certain frequency clusters are called beta waves (13 Hz and faster), theta waves (4 to 7 Hz), and alpha rhythm, a term used for waves of a sinusoidal type between 8 and 13 Hz over posterior head regions. The posterior alpha waves disappear with eye opening or certain mental tasks, and signify that a person is awake but relaxed. A similar alpha rhythm, called paradoxical alpha activity, may occur in REM sleep. The EMG recording in the waking state, even in a calm and relaxed person, contains a baseline level of tonic muscle activity in certain facial muscles, especially the mentalis muscle or occipital-cervical muscles. Brief darting eye movements or eye blinks often occur even in resting humans, always in a conjugate manner in the normal state. The states of hypnosis or meditational trance are usually accompanied by EEG patterns of wakefulness, and often will have increased alpha production.

Stage I (Drowsiness)

A person in stage I sleep behaviorally appears to be in a light sleep and may shuffle or twist slightly in bed. Onset of stage I sleep is best exemplified by the student in a lecture room. The individual's head nods slowly, the pupils constrict and dilate in a slow, fluctuating manner, the eyeballs roll slowly to and fro, and the eyelids slowly partially or completely close. If asked, the individual may say that he or she was awake although being aware of a drowsy feeling. With measurement of reaction times to stimuli or other testing of responsiveness, it can easily be demonstrated that response times and intellectual acuity are diminished, although the individual may not be aware of this drop. He or she may feel fully attentive to surrounding activity and yet objective observers will note diminished responsiveness.

   The polygraphic signs of stage I sleep consist of the disappearance of alpha rhythm, gradual suppression of overall EEG voltage, and usually subsequent emergence of diffuse 4-1 to 7-Hz low-voltage theta activity (Figure 4.1). Often, particularly in persons ingesting barbiturates, benzodiazepines, or chloral hydrate, there are clusters or spindles of rhythmical 15- to 25-Hz beta waves bifrontally or around the vertex. Although some EEG texts say that alpha rhythm slows with drowsiness, the alpha frequency seldom falls

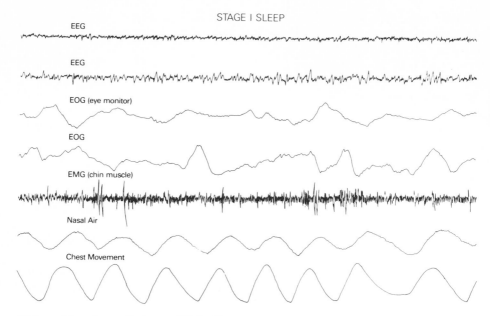

Figure 4.1. Stage I sleep. EEG (first two lines) shows disappearance of alpha rhythm, gradual development of theta wave frequencies, and voltages of 50 to 100 μV. Among the most reliable signs at the onset of stage I sleep are the slow, rolling eye movements demonstrated in the third and fourth channels. The chin EMG generally shows slight relaxation from the waking state, and respirations for the most part are regular and unlabored.

below 8 Hz in normal individuals even when drowsy. The alpha rhythm should usually disappear before the EEG is overtaken by slow waves.

The most reliable sign of this stage is not truly in the EEG, but in the eyes. With pupillometry, a slow, conjugate constriction and dilation of the pupils occurs at one- to three-second intervals as an individual nods into stage I, together with slow random movements of the eyes in somewhat circular movements that may be disconjugate. These movements occur under closed lids or as the lids slowly droop in a person "falling asleep." In the sleep laboratory, electrodes are conventionally placed above or lateral to the eyes. The electrical dipole of the corneoretinal axis causes a large electrical field, which reflects in slow, undulating lines on the polygraph paper the slow, rolling eye movements. Either DC or AC amplifiers with very slow time constant are necessary to demonstrate maximally such slow movements.

The eye movements of stage I sleep are virtually impossible to reproduce consciously. Tracking eye movements of the occipitocerebellar pathways in wakefulness give rise to slow eye movements, but not in a random manner, and often there are interspersed saccades, or rapid eye movements, between slow movement portions. Volitional eye movements are of a more rapid and small-excursion type, and so persons trying to reproduce the slow rolling eye movements of drowsiness usually have some brief, more rapid movements interspersed.

Stage II

This is the phase in which consciousness is altered enough that most people, if awakened, usually recognize having been "asleep." Yet often, as in stage I, subjects may maintain enough awareness of the environment that when awakened they do not realize the degree to which consciousness was blunted. Although some perceptual distortions and simple fantasies may occur during state I (daydreams), it is only with stage II sleep that dreams of an integrated story or plot line first become noticeable. Dream recall is far less vivid than in REM, and dreams appear to lack colorful symbolic imagery in stage II sleep, although they do occur in this stage.

Body movement is diminished somewhat and thresholds to arousal by tactile stimulation, speech, or body movement are somewhat higher in this stage. As in all levels of sleep, the stimuli necessary for arousal are lighter when they have significance for the individual. For example, nonsense syllables or meaningless words require much greater sound intensity to awaken an individual from stage II sleep than do words with emotional impact such as the subject's name.

Three main EEG patterns characterize onset of stage II sleep. Most consistent of these is the sleep spindle, also called sigma activity or sigma waves by electroencephalographers.

Electroencephalographers at times quibble about terminology. Many rhythmical waveforms produce a form on paper resembling spindles of yarn or string. The word spindle when used to describe EEG forms conveys such a specific image to many that it is confined only to sleep spindles. This may be an unfortunate restriction of a descriptive term, but at least it is useful to know how the word is used in its narrowest sense in order to avoid confusion in discussing EEG forms.

The arrival of spindles is considered to be the onset of sleep in conventional diagnostic EEG recording, and in fact most active sleep laboratories define sleep latency, or the beginning of sleep, as the time after lights are turned off until onset of the first spindle. Spindles are rhythmical clusters of 40- to 100-μV waves with frequencies ranging from 10 to 16 Hz, and lasting 0.5 to 3 seconds or occasionally longer. As with all brain waves, amplitude or voltage of waveforms vary greatly among individuals and also according to the electrode montage or connections used for recording. Hence voltage intensity is seldom an important criterion in sleep recording, unless there should be an asymmetry over the two hemispheres. Spindle distribution is bilateral, being rather wide in the frontocentral regions of the scalp (Figure 4.2). Spindles are always symmetrical beyond 6 months of age, and

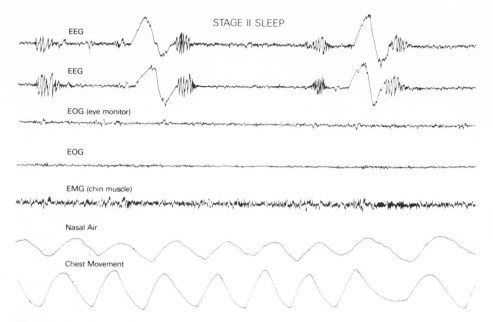

Figure 4.2.   Stage II sleep. This stage is sometimes called spindle sleep because of the occurrence of 12- to 16-Hz (cycles per second) sharp spindle waveforms best seen in paracentral regions symmetrically. These rapid bursts of rhythmical sharp waves are sometimes called sigma waves, and can be noted four times in channels 1 and 2 above. Another characteristic of stage II sleep are high-voltage (often higher than 200 μV) and blunted biphasic waveforms called K-complexes, shown above preceding the second and between the third and fourth sleep spindles. Eye movements are usually quiet during stage II sleep, and the EMG frequently shows slight diminution compared to stage I. Respirations remain regular and often shallower than in stage I sleep.

when unilateral or asynchronous over the hemispheres, they indicate cerebral dysfunction. A time-honored sign of thalamic or hemispheric dysfunction in clinical EEG is the suppression of spindles over one hemisphere.

Spindles may be elicited in the sleeping individual by a wide range of stimuli. They begin in the earliest stages of stage II sleep in a less regular manner and with frequencies that may be as slow as 12 to 13 Hz. After stage II has been more clearly developed for 5 to 15 minutes, spindles become more regular and rhythmical, and more clearly defined from the background EEG activity. They often are more visible and more intense and frequent in occurrence just before the onset of a REM interval.

Another characteristic pattern of stage II sleep, which occurs to some degree in deeper stage I sleep, are the vertex sharp waves or V waves. Vertex waves, like spindles, are triggered to some degree by stimuli, but also like spindles, can occur as often as every 30 seconds without a notable stimulus. Hence vertex waves seem to represent a nonspecific arousal pattern. They have a surface-negative polarity just at the vertex and in an area spread only a few centimeters from the vertex. Inasmuch as the field of distribution on the scalp is rather restricted, if the recording electrodes are placed in disadvantageous positions or are widely spaced, vertex waves may not be recorded at all. Vertex sharp waves are particularly prominent in children, and among children and adolescents they may recur at rapid intervals for 20 to 30 seconds on occasion, causing an appearance that suggests electrographic seizures to the naive observer.

A high-voltage (often greater than 100 μV) slow wave with a field of distribution in the frontocentral region is called a K-complex. This sharpened, moundlike waveform has an initial surface-negative (upward deflection) wave, the entire complex sometimes occupying more than one second. These K-complexes may have bilateral fields of maximum, so that appropriate recording techniques may render an appearance of independent waveforms in both the left and right frontocentral regions. The K-complexes are specifically elicited by auditory stimuli, and often coincide with generalized body twitches or myoclonic jerks of one lower extremity.

Both K-complexes and vertex waves may precede or coincide with sleep spindles. Noting this coincidence, some authors have given the misleading, probably unfortunate, name K-complex to the coincidence of vertex sharp wave and spindles. Although the precise behavioral and physiological significance of these three forms is somewhat uncertain, and all seem to represent a type of cerebral response to internally or externally generated arousals, they are certainly distinguishable. The vertex wave in particular has a clearly different field of distribution from K-complexes and spindles.

Stages III and IV (Slow Wave Sleep)

The stage of sleep characterized by the most striking degree of immobility, or which appears to be deepest in terms of resistance to arousal, is characterized by high-voltage slow waves or delta waves on EEG (Figure 4.3). Hence this phase of sleep is often called delta sleep or deep sleep. The transition between stage II and slow wave sleep is often subtle and hard to define, because spindles may persist even as slow wave sleep develops, and because K-complexes (which after all are a form of high-voltage slow waves) may become gradually more prevalent, then virtually confluent, and then merge almost imperceptibly into continuous slow waves.

Slow wave sleep is the stage that varies most with age. People beyond the age of 60 years may have virtually no slow wave sleep, and very young children have many high-voltage slow waves even with the lightest phases of drowsiness. This is also the phase that is most responsive or vulnerable to changes of activity, as discussed in Chapters 2 and 3.

There are quantitative changes of the voltage, frequency spectrum, and power spectrum of slow waves within slow wave sleep. Stage III sleep

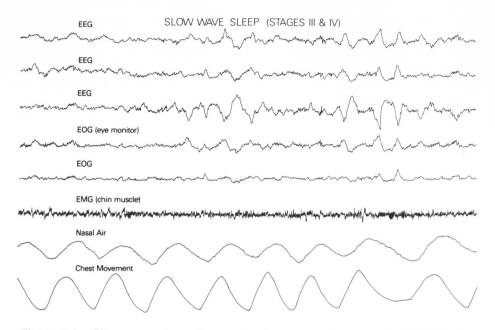

Figure 4.3. Slow wave sleep. Formerly, slow wave sleep was divided into two different classifications, depending on the duration and voltage of slow waves seen during a particular epoch of the recording. The characteristics of slow wave sleep are disappearance of sleep spindles and emergence and coalescence of slow waves on the EEG. Often the transition from stage II to slow wave sleep may be quite subtle, and seem simply to be the merging of many high-voltage K-complexes. Eye movements are usually absent, but since the eye monitor electrodes are placed near the front of the brain, high-voltage frontal delta waves are often recorded by the electrodes used for monitoring eye movement. Respirations remain slow and regular, and muscle tone is not significantly changed from stage II sleep.

is defined (Rechtschaffen and Kales, 1968) as an EEG epoch "in which at least 20 percent but not more than 50 percent of the epoch consists of waves of 2 CPS (Hz) or slower which have amplitudes greater than 75 microvolts from peak to peak." As mentioned, amplitude is a somewhat misleading criterion for any EEG wave, because it varies greatly even in healthy persons, and as written by an EEG or polygraph, is in large measure a function of the montage or sequence of electrode connections on the scalp.

Stage IV sleep is defined by an EEG recording "in which 50 percent of the epoch consists of waves of 2 CPS or slower which have amplitudes greater than 75 microvolts peak to peak." This distinction between the stages appears to be somewhat arbitrary. Although the responsiveness to most arousal stimuli is diminished in approximate proportion to the intensity of delta activity, and the greater prevalence of delta waves generally represents a deeper form of slow wave sleep, the transition between 20 percent presence of delta waves and total EEG spectrum of delta activity seems to be a continuum. Therefore, although the distinctions between wakefulness, stage I, stage II, slow wve, and REM sleep all seem to be qualitative and represent clearly distinguishable signs of physiological differences, the distinction between stages III and IV seems arbitrary. To be sure, using techniques such as spectral analysis there is a behavioral and physiological distinction between the lighter or "less delta" phases of stage III and the deeper phases of stage IV, but in terms of qualitative biological states the distinction is probably not warranted. In this book, stages III and IV usually are considered together as slow wave sleep.

Rapid Eye Movement Sleep (Dream State)

The term *paradoxical* was first used to describe the active form of sleep during which eye movements or body twitches occurred in laboratory mammals. The EEG appears to be desynchronized as a waking animal, and yet the animal appears to be deeply asleep. In humans, this electrographic pattern usually emerges from a stage II epoch. The two features noted earliest by investigators of sleep physiology were that the EEG patterns resembled those of stage I because the voltage was lower than in stage II or slow wave sleep, and the frequency spectrum seemed to be a random or nonrhythmical pattern with mixed frequencies between 4 and 25 Hz. A pattern of saw-toothed waves was often noted around the vertex or in temporal regions, consisting of slightly rhythmical, sharp, 25- to 40-μV waves. Alpha rhythm only rarely occurred in the posterior head region, just as in wakefulness. Most striking to early investigators were bursts of rapid eye movements that could be noted by simply watching the individual. These consisted of conjugate, rapidly darting movements of the eyes under closed lids in all directions of gaze, most often laterally. In fact, the eye movements were of a jerking saccadic or nystagmoid type seldom reproducible volitionally. They occurred in brief clusters lasting 3 to 10 seconds, at intervals of 30 to 40 seconds.

The behavioral state and EEG pattern characterizing this phase may at times occur without rapid eye movements at all. This may happen particularly in the first REM epoch of the night in anybody, but some individuals seldom have eye movements in REM. The most reliable sign of REM or active sleep is the disappearance of tonic somatic muscle activity. The individual becomes more limp than at any other time, and tonic muscle activity, usually recorded under the jaw or on the mentalis muscle, disappears (Figure 4.4). By noting the EMG channel, the somnographer then is able to notice the occurrence of REM sleep without eye movements. Other features occur during REM sleep such as fluctuations in blood pressure, irregular respirations, irregular pulse rate, perspiration, premature ventricular contractions, penile erections, and increased vaginal secretion.

Dreams recalled during REM sleep, especially in the later stages of

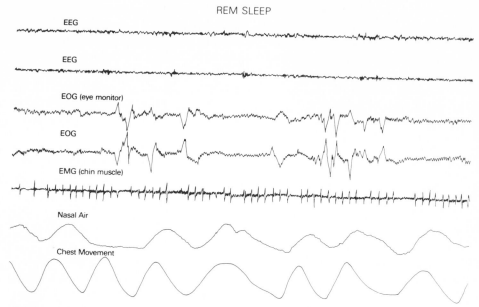

Figure 4.4. Rapid eye movement (REM, paradoxical) sleep. In REM sleep, the EEG patterns resemble either wakefulness or stage I sleep. The eye movements occur in quick, conjugate, darting bursts at intervals of 4 to 10 seconds. The somatic EMG flattens, that is, diminishes. In this example, the chin electrodes show a flattening of the EMG but heuristically also record the ECG, and demonstrate one of the other characteristics of REM sleep: the irregular pulse that occurs in some individuals. Respirations may become quite irregular, as demonstrated here, with some partial obstruction at the upper airway so that chest movements are not always accompanied by air exchange at the mouth or nose. REM sleep usually develops, or rather emerges, from stage II sleep, rather than progressing from slow wave sleep.

the night, are more complex, vivid, and erotic than those in other stages. Arousal thresholds to most stimuli are lower during REM sleep than in slow wave sleep.

Because the EEG pattern of REM sleep superficially resembles that of stage I, REM is sometimes called stage I REM. In fact, the EEG spectrum of REM sleep usually has a somewhat higher frequency distribution and the general EEG voltage or power is lower than in stage I sleep. Similarly, the disappearance of somatic muscle tone during REM and the slow rolling eye movements of stage I sleep separate these two stages. The arousal thresholds to most stimuli are higher in REM sleep. For the most part, it is probably incorrect to consider that REM and stage I sleep are part of the same physiological level. For this reason, in this book REM is considered a separate stage, not a special stage of stage I. Conventional sleep stage histograms also plot REM with stage I, but we plot them separately.

Characteristics on EEG of REM sleep actually most nearly resemble background EEG patterns seen in stage II sleep if K-complexes, vertex waves, and spindles are excluded. In fact, it is intriguing that REM phases usually emerge from stage II sleep.

Different Stages and Depth of Sleep

Common experience is to recognize that some phases of sleep are more satisfying or that individuals are more difficult to arouse at different times of the night. Hence when different physiological states are definable for the phenomenon of sleep, it is tempting to speak in terms of depth of sleep or to imply that the various stages represent a graded intensity. This is misleading because a recurring sequence in the pattern of nocturnal sleep really suggests specific physiological functions for each stage rather than a range or depth of a single one. It may be that early investigators expected that depth or satiety of sleep would correlate with various EEG patterns. Perhaps it would have been more useful to invoke terminology such as theta sleep for stage I, spindle sleep for stage II, and slow wave sleep (a term often used now) for stages III and IV, and to continue the descriptive terminology rather than to use numbers or graphs with higher and lower levels to depict stages.

Florida Laboratory Criteria

Not all laboratories use the scoring and terminology system of Rechtschaffen and Kales. One other scheme was developed by the University of Florida laboratory and reported by Williams, Karacan, and Hursch (1974). Use of these criteria resulted in more than 90 percent concurrence when the recordings were interpreted at different times or by different reviewers.

Stage 0   The condition of wakefulness before sleep begins, defined by a minimum of 30 seconds of 8- to 12-Hz occipital activity (alpha waves) with amplitude of at least 40 μV peak to peak.

Stage 1   Less than 30 seconds of alpha rhythm and not more than 1 well-defined sleep spindle or K-complex. If no clear alpha rhythm was noted while awake, then disappearance of muscle artifact or eye movements is used to determine onset.

Stage 2   At least 2 well-defined sleep spindles or K-complexes; not more than 12 seconds of delta waves.

Stage 3   At least 13 seconds of 1- to 3-Hz, 40 μV slow waves, but less than 30 seconds of this activity.

Stage 4   Differs from stage 3 by presence of more than 30 dominant seconds of high-voltage delta waves (1- to 3-Hz, above 40-μV) in every minute.

These criteria are for scoring minute by minute during sleep.

NORMAL NOCTURNAL SLEEP SEQUENCE

The normal sequence of sleep varies with age, with diurnal activity, and with physical and emotional environment. Among healthy young adults there are 32 stage changes in an average night in the laboratory, but even this sequence varies as the subject becomes accustomed to the sleeping environment. The so-called first-night effect (Agnew, Wilse, and Williams, 1966) prolongs sleep latency, shortens total sleep time (TST) and REM time, and shows how sensitive or adaptive the sleep sequence is in response to environmental manipulation. One of the most authoritative studies of the normal sleep cycle was reported by Williams, Karacan, and Hursch in 1974. They studied characteristics of sleep in 243 healthy individuals, equal numbers of females and males at all ages up to 70 years (Table 4.1).

In an appropriate environment, in a comfortable bed and darkened room, the average individual between ages 3 and 80 years lapses into stage I sleep within seven minutes, sometimes slower in the elderly; the latency to stage II, or the appearance of the first sleep spindles, ranges from five to nine minutes at virtually all ages, with no persistent difference between males and females (Williams, Karacan, and Hursch, 1974). For young adults, the first slow wave sleep epoch usually begins 30 minutes thereafter and lasts 15 to 30 minutes. For children under the age of 9, the onset of slow wave sleep appears an average of 10 minutes after the beginning of stage II. By contrast, the average latency to the onset of slow wave sleep for persons beyond 50 years of age is 55 minutes. For the most part, the sequence or cycle of sleep stages averages about 90 minutes, varying greatly with age. Except for REM onset, sleep is less intense or less efficient in the elderly (Figure 4.6). The latency to onset of the first REM is briefest in old age, averaging 85 minutes for persons over 50, 90 minutes for those between the ages of 20 and 49 years, and 120 minutes for children under the age of 9. Older people sleep less than young people, with an average total sleep time of 400 minutes in people over the age of 50, but an average of 420 minutes for those between the ages of 20 and 50, and 520 minutes for children and adolescents. Children under the age of 9 average seven rapid eye movement cycles, whereas people over 50 years of age average only four. The number of awakenings is predictably higher among people over 50, averaging seven per night, whereas children and adolescents awaken an average of one to three times per night. Young adults between the ages of 20 and 49 years average four awakenings per night for males and two for females.

As shown in Figure 4.5, slow wave sleep predominates in the first half

Table 4.1. Normative Sleep Data in 243 Volunteers of Several Ages

	Age 9 and Under	Age 10–19	Age 20–49	Over 50
Time in bed (M/F)	606/615	515/510	435/443	456/480
Total sleep time (M/F)	620/580	500/510	410/427	390/416
Sleep latency	16 ± 7.5	17.5 ± 9	10 ± 9	22 ± 20
Sleep period time (M/F) from first sleep to final arousal	560/570	500/510	423/432	432/456
SPT spent awake (%)	1/1	2/1	3/2	9/9
SPT spent in stage I (%)	2/2	2/3	6/5	9/7
SPT spent in stage II (%)	48/48	50/50	50/50	58/55
SPT spent in stages III and IV (%)	21/21	23/22	14/15	3/10
SPT spent in REM (%)	29/31	25/25	29/26	21/21
Once asleep, latency to stage II	——— No change with age; 5–9 minutes ———			
Once asleep, latency to SWS (III)	10/10	15/15	30/30	55/45
Once asleep, REM latency (sleep onset to REM onset)	120/120	110/110	90/90	85/85
Number of REM periods per night	7/7	5/5	4/4	4/4
Average length of REM period	30/30	28/28	29/29	22/23
Number of nocturnal awakenings	1/1	3/2	4/2	7/6

From Williams, Karacan, and Hursch (1974).

of the night and REM periods become longer as the night goes on, so that the bulk of REM sleep occurs in the later half.

At all ages, stage II sleep accounts for 50 percent or more of total sleep time, and REM sleep usually arises from stage II. The typical sequence of gradual progression from stage I, stage II, slow wave sleep, and then back to stage II precedes onset of any REM epoch, even though the pre-REM stage II phase may last only one or two minutes. Periods of body immobility lasting 30 minutes or longer occur mostly in association with slow wave sleep or descending stage II: stage II with prominent slow waves or just before onset of slow wave sleep (Hobson, Spagna, Malenka, 1978). When subjects are asked to comment upon the "goodness" of sleep or a

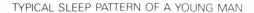

TYPICAL SLEEP PATTERN OF A YOUNG MAN

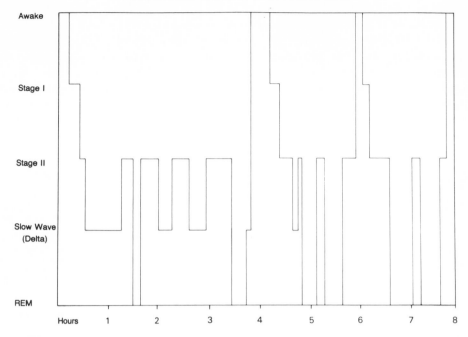

Figure 4.5. Typical sleep pattern of a young man. Note the onset of sleep (stage I) within 15 minutes after lights are turned out. Slow wave sleep predominates in the first half of the night, and REM sleep occurs more consistently and intensely in the second half. REM intervals recur at approximately 90-minute intervals, although they have a longer duration in the second half of the night. There are only two nocturnal awakenings. REM sleep, which consumes 20 to 25 percent of the total night's sleep, almost always emerges from stage II sleep. Total sleep time is approximately 6.5 to 8 hours.

sense of satiety either because of physical relaxation or sense of well being after sleep, such reports best correlate with the duration of immobility times or with awakening directly from immobility periods.

Arousal Thresholds to Determine Sleep Levels

Almost intuitively, people recognize different degrees of responsiveness or arousal from sleep, which of course leads to the colloquial concept of depth of sleep. Although there is a very rough correlation between the intensity of stimulus required to awaken a person and sleep stages numbered I through IV, this correlation is quite variable (Okuma, Nakamura, Hayashi, et al, 1966; Lester, 1958; Steriade, Iosif, and Apostol, 1969; Zung and Wilson, 1961). In fact, there are generally two repetitive "troughs" of arousal thresholds in many subjects that are virtually superimposed upon the sleep stage sequence. At least for auditory stimuli, REM sleep often has the highest threshold, that is, requires the greatest intensity of stimulus, to auditory arousal (Zung and Wilson, 1961; Williams, Karacan, and Hursch, 1974). This threshold is different, however, for pure tones or loud noises than for language. For example, words or comments of significance or with emotional content are far more effective as arousal stimuli than pure tones during REM. The comment, "John, it is time to get up now," is likely to awaken a person from his final REM period, and a statement that "The house is on fire" is almost certain to awaken an individual. By contrast, comments with erotic implications or that can fit into a story line may be incorporated into a dream during REM and not awaken the individual at all. For these reasons, arousal threshold is not a reliable predictor of quality of sleep stages, at least as they are defined electrophysiologically.

The commonly used criteria for staging sleep sequence have obviously evolved because of the accessibility or convenience of patterns that occur in most mammals and virtually all humans. This schema is reasonably consistent and certainly provides a group of things to measure. The lack of correlation between arousal thresholds, the permeation of dreams into all of the various sleep stages, and the uncertainty about the biological significance of these stages for the organism are among the inadequacies of current classifications.

Perhaps a graver criticism of the current scheme of staging sleep is the general lack of transition phases. Few biological stages vary by abrupt flip-flop to a totally different qualitative stage. This is particularly true with altered states of consciousness. Certainly, the transition from wakefulness to drowsiness and sleep is a gradual one; people usually recognize when they change from full wakefulness to drowsiness. Similarly, the fact that full alertness evolves gradually after awakening rather than immediately is evidence that awakening is not an instantaneous process. This obtains as well for changes in levels of alertness in pathological states: after seizures there is a period of postictal neurological depression; before the loss of consciousness in syncope there is a period of lipothymia, or lightheadedness; in metabolic states giving rise to coma, there is a gradual transition to loss of consciousness. With analysis of the spectrum of frequencies and scalp electrical power voltage, it is clear that there are transitions among sleep stages. For example, between stages II and III (slow wave sleep), the proliferation of K-complexes and gradual blending of continuous delta waves often occur as a transition phase. Sleep spindles often persist into the early stages of stage III, and in some older individuals, spindles persist throughout slow wave sleep as they do in certain pathological conditions such as Parkinson's disease.

Depiction of sleep stages in typical histograms or graphs implies more abrupt transitions between the levels of sleep than is probably physiologically correct. It is important to recognize the arbitrary nature of sleep stages and the nature of their occurrence.

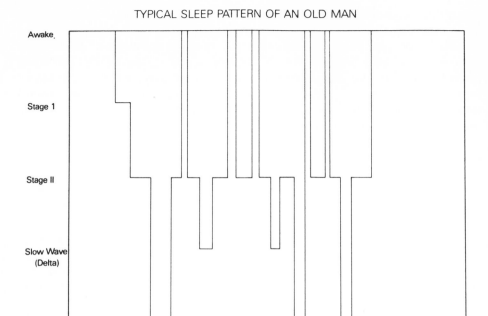

Figure 4.6. Note that sleep onset is slower than in youth, in this individual being nearly one hour. There is much less slow wave sleep, occurring less often and for shorter periods. REM sleep still consumes 20 to 25 percent of total sleep time, but since this time is only about six hours, total REM is less. There are five nocturnal awakenings and the cyclicity of REM sleep is less apparent.

Normative Data on Sleep Patterns

As discussed by Ferber in Chapter 6, the sequence and characteristics of sleep in the infant and child differ from those in the adult, and with aging sleep characteristics change. There is very little difference in the quality or duration of sleep between the sexes, however. In a study of 243 patients, Williams, Karacan, and Hursch (1974) compiled normative data for the duration and sequence of sleep stages at several ages, and compared males to females. Some of the basic characteristics are presented in Table 4.1. The amount of time spent in bed decreases throughout life until the sixth and seventh decades, when it increases somewhat. Total sleep time, however, continues to decrease throughout life, so that the amount of time spent in bed awake increases from only 1 percent of the total sleep period time in children to 9 percent or more among the elderly. The most conspicuous decline occurs in slow wave sleep, occupying more than 20 percent of the sleep period time (SPT) for people under the age of 19, 3 percent in males beyond the age of 50, and 10 percent among females beyond the age of 50. The percentage of SPT spent in REM, by contrast, does not decline to a significant degree with age, although the absolute duration of REM does diminish proportionately with the decline in SPT. The number of REM periods declines from an average of seven among people under the age of 9 years to five or fewer in persons beyond the age of 20, and sometimes only two REM spells among the elderly. The average number of nocturnal awakenings is only one among children, but increases to seven among males beyond the age of 50 years. In other words, the intensity, duration, and continuity of sleep all diminish with age. Slow wave sleep in particular occurs less often with age, as do the number and duration of REM epochs. Proportionately, there is also an increase in the number of nocturnal awakenings with older age.

REFERENCES

Agnew H, Wilse B, Williams R. The first night effect—an EEG study of sleep. Psychophysiology 1966;2:263–66.

Dement WC, Kleitman N. The relation of eye movements during sleep to dream activity: an objective method for the study of dreaming. J Exp Psychol 1957;53:339–46.

Guilleminault WC. Sleeping and waking disorders: indications and techniques. Menlo Park, Calif.: Addison-Wesley, 1982.

Hobson JA, Spagna T, Malenka R. Ethology of sleep studied with time-lapse photography: postural immobility and sleep-cycle phase in humans. Science 1978;201:1251–53.

Lester D. Continuous measurement of the depth of sleep. Science 1958;127:1340–41.

Loomis AL, Harvey EN, Hobart GA. Cerebral states during sleep as studied by human brain potentials. J Exp Physiol 1937;21:127–44.

Okuma T, Nakamura K, Hayashi A, Fujimori M. Psychophysiological study of the depth of sleep in normal human subjects. Electroencephalogr Clin Neurophysiol 1966;21:140–47.

Rechtschaffen A, Kales A. A manual of standardized terminology: techniques and scoring for sleep stages of human subjects. NIH Publication no. 204. Bethesda, Md.: National Institutes of Health, 1968.

Steriade M, Iosif G, Apostol V. Responsiveness of thalamic and cortical motor replays during arousal and various stages of sleep. J Neurophysiol 1969;32:251–65.

Williams RL, Karacan I, Hursch CJ. Electroencephalography of human sleep: clinical applications. New York: John Wiley & Sons, 1974.

Zung WW, Wilson WP. Response to auditory stimulation during sleep. Discrimination and arousal as studied with electroencephalography. Arch Gen Psychiatry 1961;4:548–52.

PART II

Abnormal Sleep

CHAPTER 5

Primary Sleep Disorders and Insomnia
Peter J. Hauri

This chapter is written from the sleep clinician's point of view, focusing on insomnia, excessive daytime sleepiness, disorders of the sleep-wake schedule, and finally, the parasomnias, that is, the dysfunctions associated with sleep, sleep stages, and partial arousals. Issues of diagnosis and treatment are covered for each of these pathologies. There is also some suggestion about when to refer these patients to a sleep disorders center.

Until 20 years ago, sleep researchers were basic scientists, interested mainly in theory and in shedding some light on the mechanisms of sleep, its physiology, and psychology. This has changed. By about 1970 enough knowledge had accumulated on sleep to become clinically useful. A whole new field of sleep disorders medicine sprang up and was practiced in specialized centers. By 1975 enough of these centers had developed to form the Association of Sleep Disorders Centers (ASDC). This association attempts to maintain standards among its member centers by offering educational opportunities, certification of centers that meet standards, and examinations of the sleep clinicians (somnologists) who work in them. (Information about certified centers may be obtained from the Association of Sleep Disorders Centers, Office of the Secretary/Treasurer, P.O. Box 2604, Del Mar, CA 92014.)

One achievement of the ASDC was the development of a formal nosology for all sleep disorders (Association of Sleep Disorders Centers, 1979) (Table 5.1). While this nosology has little official standing, there are recommended ICD 9-CM codes, and it is hoped that a modified version of it will be officially incorporated into ICD 10.

For the sleep clinician, the basic tool is still the all-night recording of sleep on the polygraph, called a somnogram (see Chapter 9). A somnogram should always be obtained during the hours when a patient would typically sleep at home. Usually a technician monitors the polygraph throughout the night, while a two-way intercom maintains voice contact with the patient.

Obviously, recording patients for entire nights is expensive. This has led many clinicians to use the more subjective evaluation of sleep distur-

Table 5.1.   Outline of Diagnostic Classification of Sleep and Arousal Disorders

A.   DIMS: Disorders of initiating and maintaining sleep (insomnias)
   1. Psychophysiological
      a. Transient and situational
      b. Persistent
   2. Associated with psychiatric disorders
      a. Symptom and personality disorders
      b. Affective disorders
      c. Other functional psychoses
   3. Associated with use of drugs and alcohol
      a. Tolerance to or withdrawal from CNS depressants
      b. Sustained use of CNS stimulants
      c. Sustained use of or withdrawal from other drugs
      d. Chronic alcoholism
   4. Associated with sleep-induced respiratory impairment
      a. Sleep apnea DIMS syndrome
      b. Alveolar hypoventilation DIMS syndrome
   5. Associated with sleep-related (nocturnal) myoclonus and restless legs
      a. Sleep-related (nocturnal) myoclonus DIMS syndrome
      b. Restless legs DIMS syndrome
   6. Associated with other medical, toxic, and environmental conditions
   7. Childhood-onset DIMS
   8. Associated with other DIMS conditions
      a. Repeated REM sleep interruptions
      b. Atypical polysomnographic features
      c. Not otherwise specified*
   9. No DIMS abnormality
      a. Short sleeper
      b. Subjective DIMS complaint without objective findings
      c. Not otherwise specified*
B.   DOES: Disorders of excessive somnolence
   1. Psychophysiological
      a. Transient and situational
      b. Persistent
   2. Associated with psychiatric disorders
      a. Affective disorders
      b. Other functional disorders
   3. Associated with use of drugs and alcohol
      a. Tolerance to or withdrawal from CNS stimulants
      b. Sustained use of CNS depressants
   4. Associated with sleep-induced respiratory impairment
      a. Sleep apnea DOES syndrome
      b. Alveolar hypoventilation DOES syndrome
   5. Associated with sleep-related (nocturnal) myoclonus and restless legs
      a. Sleep-related (nocturnal) myoclonus DOES syndrome
      b. Restless legs DOES syndrome
   6. Narcolepsy
   7. Idiopathic CNS hypersomnolence
   8. Associated with other medical, toxic, and environmental conditions

Table 5.1.   *(continued)*

9. Associated with other DOES conditions
    a. Intermittent DOES (periodic) syndromes
        i. Kleine-Levin syndrome
        ii. Menstrual-associated syndrome
    b. Insufficient sleep
    c. Sleep drunkenness
    d. Not otherwise specified*
10. No DOES abnormality
    a. Long sleeper
    b. Subjective DOES complaint without objective findings
    c. Not otherwise specified*

C. Disorders of the sleep-wake schedule
    1. Transient
        a. Rapid time zone change (jet lag) syndrome
        b. Work shift change in conventional sleep-wake schedule
    2. Persistent
        a. Frequently changing sleep-wake schedule
        b. Delayed sleep phase syndrome
        c. Advanced sleep phase syndrome
        d. Non-24-hour sleep-wake syndrome
        e. Irregular sleep-wake pattern
        f. Not otherwise specified*

D. Dysfunctions associated with sleep, sleep stages, or partial arousals (parasomnias)
    1. Sleepwalking (somnambulism)
    2. Sleep terror (pavor nocturnus, incubus)
    3. Sleep-related enuresis
    4. Other dysfunctions
        a. Dream anxiety attacks (nightmares)
        b. Sleep-related epileptic seizures
        c. Sleep-related bruxism
        d. Sleep-related head banging (jactatio capitis nocturnus)
        e. Familial sleep paralysis
        f. Impaired sleep-related penile tumescence
        g. Sleep-related painful erections
        h. Sleep-related cluster headaches and chronic paroxysmal hemicrania
        i. Sleep-related abnormal swallowing syndrome
        j. Sleep-related asthma
        k. Sleep-related cardiovascular symptoms
        l. Sleep-related gastroesophageal reflux
        m. Sleep-related hemolysis (paroxysmal nocturnal hemoglobinuria)
        n. Asymptomatic polysomnographic finding
        o. Not otherwise specified*

*This entry is intended to leave place in the classification for both undiagnosed ("don't know") conditions and additional (as yet undocumented) conditions that may be described in the future.

Reprinted by permission from the Association of Sleep Disorders Centers (1979).

bances through sleep logs filled out at home and interviews with patients and bed partners. Unfortunately, these more subjective self-report data correlate quite poorly with somnograms obtained on the polygraph. Patients usually are unaware of their muscle twitches or respiratory pauses during sleep, cannot report on electroencephalographical (EEG) abnormalities during sleep, and usually underestimate the amount of sleep they get during the night.

Actually, the problem is even more complex. When awakened from polygraphically assessed, unmistakable sleep, some patients, especially some insomniacs, report that they had been awake and thinking (Borkovec, Lane, and VanOot, 1981) and can report long, bonafide trains of thoughts. It seems debatable whether such patients were asleep before the "awakening" as the polygraph suggests, or awake, as their thinking would indicate. Conversely, patients with obstructive sleep apneas may report that they have slept soundly and without awakening for 8 to 10 hours, while the polygraph may indicate hundreds of awakenings throughout the night and suggest that the patient has spent most of the night dozing or in very light sleep.

The discrepancies between subjective reports and somnograms provide much of the basis for the different approaches between general practice and work in a sleep disorders center. The sleep clinician relies on the somnogram for guidance; the general practitioner mainly treats the patient's complaint.

GENERAL SLEEP CHARACTERISTICS

Age Relationships

As Figure 5.1 indicates, age may be the most important determinant of a person's sleep (Williams, Karacan, and Hursch, 1974). Most dramatic are the changes that occur with age for delta sleep, rapid eye movement (REM) sleep, and stage I sleep (the transition between waking and sleeping). Figure 5.1 was developed on healthy sleepers. It seems important to note that after the age of 35 years, total time asleep still gradually declines while total time in bed starts to climb again. This can only mean that even healthy people spend more time lying in bed unable to sleep as they grow older.

Not only does the pattern of sleep change, but complaints about sleep change as well. Young insomniacs typically have difficulties falling alseep, but once asleep they sleep well, while older insomniacs have difficulty sleeping through the night in addition to suffering from early morning awakening. Also, older people are generally unable to remain awake all day and take frequent naps. Other problems are also age related: night terrors and sleepwalking are often seen in children, narcolepsy usually starts in the second decade, and sleep apneas increase dramatically with advancing age.

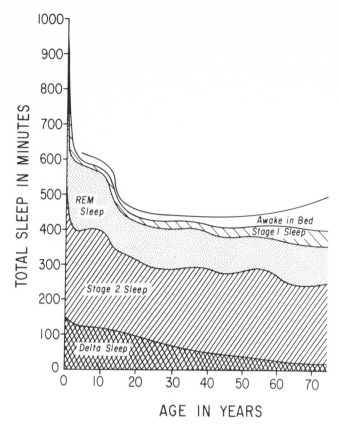

Figure 5.1. Development of sleep over a lifetime. (Reprinted by permission from John Wiley & Sons, Inc. From Williams, Karacan, and Hursch, 1974; from Hauri, 1982.)

Sleep Needs

While Figure 5.1 gives the average amount of sleep that is obtained by the different age groups, it should not be taken as a norm for all individuals. Indeed, within the same age range, some humans might sleep only 2 or 3 hours per 24 hours and still feel well (Meddis, Pearson, and Langford, 1973), while others might need to sleep 8 to 10 hours to feel rested. Similarly, while sleep needs during childhood generally decrease, as the figure indicates, there are 4-year-olds who seem to require less sleep than some 10-year-olds.

Because of the large variability of individual sleep needs, one cannot define either insomnia or excessive daytime sleepiness by a certain number of hours a person sleeps. Rather, the first question with these disorders should be, "How do you feel when you are awake?" A person who sleeps four hours but feels alert and healthy the rest of the time may simply be a short sleeper, not an insomniac. Someone who feels alert and active after ten hours of sleep but not after seven may just require more sleep, say ten hours, as a normal biological need rather than manifestation of a disorder.

Can we manipulate our sleep needs? There is some evidence that Americans now sleep about one hour less than they did before Edison developed electric lights (Webb and Agnew, 1975), and some ascribe our frenetic lifestyle to the diminished sleep time. Indeed, Mullaney et al (1977) found that by chronically and drastically curtailing sleep for over six months, they could teach young adults to seek less sleep chronically and still feel alert. The long-range effects of such curtailed sleep regimens are not known.

Sleep Deprivation

Most people have been told during childhood that it is important to obtain a "good" night's sleep each and every night. This is not so. Losing all or most of a night's slumber results in excessive sleepiness the next day and causes deterioration of mood and ability to concentrate when the task is very boring. Beyond that, it does not seem to adversely affect most areas of functioning, and it does not seem medically or psychologically harmful (Johnson, 1969; Morgan, 1974).

When total sleep deprivation continues for more than 48 hours, "mini-sleeps" start to occur. These are epochs, at first only a few seconds in duration, where bonafide sleep EEG waves appear in an otherwise awake record. During these mini-sleeps the person is unresponsive because he or she is really asleep for a few seconds. Mini-sleeps become more abundant and longer with continuing sleep deprivation. In about ten days, it becomes impossible to tell from the EEG whether the person is actually awake or asleep, even if the sleep-deprived individual is actively engaged in physical activity.

Psychomotor performance and well-being gradually decrease with the first few days of sleep deprivation. In the beginning, these decreases may be ascribed to the mini-sleeps, but after four or five days there seems to be a genuine decrease in cognitive, psychomotor, and perceptual capabilities that cannot be overcome by increased motivation (Pasnau, Naitoh, Stier, et al, 1968). Maximum disruptive effects of total sleep deprivation are usually found within two to five days. It seems possible that after this time the gradually increasing, unavoidable mini-sleeps may give the body enough rest to maintain some low level of functioning.

When recovering from sleep deprivation, there is usually first an increase in delta sleep (Kales, Tan, Kollar, et al, 1970). If an increase in REM sleep occurs, it usually awaits the second recovery night. The amount of stage II sleep that is lost during deprivation is never recovered. Also, one does not need to recover the total duration of sleep that was lost. Recovery is usually completed in two to three nights, even if previous deprivation has lasted up to ten nights.

Loss of Specific Sleep Stages

If psychomotor performance is the issue, the total amount of lost sleep is the determining factor, while the stage that is lost seems irrelevant (Johnson, 1973). This seems less true for other areas of consideration.

Depriving a person exclusively of REM sleep apparently heightens central neural excitability and energizes basic drives or weakens control over them (Vogel, 1975). When such REM deprivation is carried out in patients with endogenous depression, it has an antidepressant effect similar to that obtained by amitriptyline (Vogel, Thurmond, Gibbons, et al, 1975). It is interesting that all currently known antidepressants are also potent REM suppressants (Vogel, 1975).

Delta sleep deprivation seems to result in musculoskeletal symptoms and increased sensitivity to pain (Moldofsky, Scarisbrick, England, et al, 1975). Indeed, disturbing delta sleep in healthy subjects results in a condition similar to fibrositis, and patients with fibrositis show disturbed non-REM (NREM) sleep. These findings concerning the different effects of REM and delta deprivation suggest that delta sleep may be related to somatic recovery, while REM sleep might be connected to the recovery of higher mental function.

Sleep Hygiene

Our 24-hour sleep-wake existence is best understood as a delicate balance between two opposing systems: the wake system (basically the ascending reticular activating system, or ARAS) and a sleep-inducing system, which is intertwined with the ARAS on many levels. The ARAS is innately the stronger of the two systems, and as long as it is relatively active, there will be no sleep. The occasional nights of insomnia that most of us experience because of stress or excitement are usually related to such ARAS arousal. Evidence is accumulating, however, that many chronic and severe insomniacs do not suffer from excessive excitement (Hauri, 1981). In these cases, one might speculate that the basic balance between the waking and sleeping circuits may be slightly tilted toward wakefulness, or that the sleep-inducing circuitry in the brainstem might be somewhat weaker than it is in a good sleeper. Basic rules of sleep hygiene are summarized in the following list on page 88. These rules, all scientifically evaluated, might help people who suffer from mild forms of insomnia. However, by themselves they will not cure serious insomniacs, although they are important in the overall treatment of such patients. Also, people who are blessed with very powerful sleep systems can violate any number of these rules and still sleep well.

1. It helps to establish a regular wakeup time each morning, even if the previous night's sleep was inadequate. This time should be kept even on weekends. This will strengthen circadian cycling and improve sleep.
2. Most insomniacs stay in bed too long, much longer than good sleepers. Cutting down on time in bed will gradually deepen sleep and decrease arousals.
3. Daytime naps help some to sleep better at night, while others sleep much more poorly after them (Evans, Cook, Cohen et al, 1977). Each person should know his or her type.
4. A healthy body sleeps better than an unfit one, however, it may take some weeks before the effects of exercise are felt (Baekeland and Lasky, 1966; Griffin and Trinder, 1978).
5. Hunger disturbs sleep (Jacobs and McGinty, 1971). A light bedtime snack is suggested, e.g., cheese and crackers, warm milk, or ovaltine (Brezinova and Oswald, 1972).
6. Many poor sleepers are very sensitive to stimulants, even to cola drinks or chocolate. Caffeine takes at least eight hours to metabolize. Thus no stimulant drinks should be taken after lunch (Karacan, Thornby, Anch, et al, 1976).
7. Sleep is clearly disturbed in smokers and in those who withdraw from heavy nicotine use (Myrsten, Elgerot and Edgren, 1977; Soldatos, Kales, Scharf et al, 1980).
8. Alcohol may help persons to fall asleep easier in the evening, but it will awaken them many times during the night. Thus by the morning they will have had less sleep than they would have without alcohol (Johnson, Burdick, and Smith, 1970).
9. Occasional loud noises (e.g., an occasional truck or airplane) disturb sleep, even in those who claim that they have adapted to them (Globus, Friedmann, Cohen, et al, 1974). Soundscreening the room with a fan or air conditioner may help.
10. The temperature in the bedroom should be comfortable. Hot rooms disturb sleep, as do excessively cold rooms (Schmidt-Kessen and Kendel, 1973; Otto, 1973).

INSOMNIA

Sleep needs vary, yet some fear that they may be insomniacs when they do not get eight hours of sleep a night. When somebody complains about poor sleep, it is wise first to ask how the person feels during wakefulness. The patient who feels relatively alert and is performing well may not need help with sleep, but rather some education on sleep needs. In making this assessment, one should bear in mind that practically everybody thinks that with a little more sleep one could function even better than normal.

Insomnia Associated with Psychiatric Disturbances

Most chronic insomnia is of psychiatric origin, the result of excessive tension, chronic depression, anxiety neurosis, poststress syndrome, or incipient psychosis. In these psychiatric insomnias, it is the psychological problem that should be treated. For example, there is no use prescribing hypnotics to patients who habitually abuse themselves by accepting overloads of work and responsibility. It will be much better to work on their lifestyles and deal with the feelings of grandiosity or inferiority that make them accept superhuman burdens.

As a rule, insomniacs are repressors (Coursey and Frankel, 1977), denying emotional problems. Patients who complain only about insomnia when the physician detects an underlying psychiatric problem such as depression have already made important statements about their diagnosis and treatment. They will have difficulties seeing their problem as psychological and will push for drug therapy while resisting psychotherapy. Therefore, in such cases the physician initially may need to be much more directive and forceful in the topics to be selected for discussion than one would be with a patient who enters the office stating a psychiatric complaint. If this is not done, the entire time may be wasted exclusively discussing the insomnia.

Treating insomnias of psychiatric origin demands a diversified approach. The basic psychological maladjustment must be dealt with, but such patients are rarely willing to sit for more than 15 minutes of "psychotherapy." Stress management techniques may have to be taught and the patients may need to learn new ways of dealing with the daily problems of living. As sleep hygiene and lifestyle issues are confronted, the patient may need to learn relaxation in the evening, do the "work of worrying" at a predetermined place and time other than in bed at night, increase exercise, regularize bedtime, and so on. Such treatment takes time. Sedating antidepressants or antipsychotics may become part of the overall treatment, or one may prescribe an occasional hypnotic to be taken no more than once or twice per week for "catch-up" sleep.

Treatment of insomnia usually is not just a matter of resolving some psychiatric problem or teaching sleep hygiene. Rather, it involves actively teaching new lifestyles and how to resolve conflicts.

Medical Insomnias

About 15 to 20 percent of chronic insomnias are secondary to medical disorders such as chronic pain, allergies, metabolic disease, and so on. Others are secondary to drugs, including alcohol. In addition, there are six medical problems that manifest themselves only in sleep and must be ruled out if insomnia persists.

Sleep-induced (Nocturnal) Myoclonus

Nocturnal myoclonus is a repetitive twitch of the legs (most easily recorded from the anterior tibialis) that occurs in regular intervals of 20 to 60 seconds. Periods of twitching last from a few minutes to several hours and alternate with periods of normal sleep, that is, without twitching. Sometimes both legs twitch, sometimes either one twitches alone. Often, these twitches are followed by signs of EEG arousal such as a K-complex or some alpha intrusion, and occasionally they awaken the sleeper.

Nocturnal myoclonus is not related to the hypnagogic twitch that some of us experience on occasion while falling asleep. Insomniacs with nocturnal myoclonus are usually unaware that they twitch, but report that they are restless sleepers, that their bedding is often very disturbed in the morning, or that bed partners have complained about their kicking. While myoclonus is found in about 12 percent of insomniacs (Coleman, 1982), many good sleepers may also show sleep-related myoclonus when monitored in the laboratory (Kales, Bixler, Soldatos, et al, 1982). Thus nocturnal myoclonus per se may not be the issue. Rather, it may become a cause of insomnia either when the twitches are severe enough to disturb sound sleep or when the patient constitutionally is a light sleeper and therefore aroused even by mild twitches.

Some cases of sleep-related myoclonus have been associated with chronic uremia or other metabolic disease. Others are found in patients treated with tricyclic antidepressants or in those recovering from use of a variety of drugs, including central nervous system (CNS) depressants. Also, the incidence increases with age, and the problem may be found frequently in those troubled by other sleep disorders such as narcolepsy or sleep apnea.

If disturbing to sleep, nocturnal myoclonus is suppressed with clonazepam, usually starting at 0.5 mg at bedtime (Coleman, 1982; Zorick, Roth, Salis, et al, 1978). Patients readily habituate to this medication, however, and then need to be withdrawn for "drug holidays" before the suppressing is reinstituted.

Restless Legs Syndrome

The restless legs syndrome is not really a sleep disorder, but a problem during relaxed wakefulness that prevents sleep (Coleman, 1982). Uncomfortable but not really painful sensations in calf and thighs disturb the patient when relaxing and disappear with walking. "When I sit down and relax, it feels like small worms crawl in my calf and thighs," reported a recent sufferer. Telling this to her physician, she was promptly admitted to a psychiatric ward for her "somatic delusions" before an alert psychiatrist diagnosed the restless legs syndrome.

This condition must be differentiated from the agitation of anxiety and stress. It has been associated with caffeinism (Lutz, 1978); motoneuron disease (Frankel, Patten, and Gillin, 1974); and poor circulation, iron deficiency, and lack of vitamins or folate. Diseases such as uremia, diabetes, carcinoma, and acute poliomyelitis have also been associated with this problem, which is often aggravated during pregnancy, but disappears with fever (Coleman, 1982). Painful polyneuropathies may especially cause this syndrome. The perplexing fact is that, unfortunately, for most patients an etiology cannot be discovered. Also, in the laboratory, the restless legs syndrome is often associated with nocturnal myoclonus, although the two may exist independently of each other.

Once the possibly associated medical diseases and deficiencies have been excluded, the restless legs syndrome can often be temporarily ameliorated with oxycodone, carbamazepine, or 5-hydroxytryptophan. Again, "drug holidays" may be needed. Some claim that an adequate exercise program will help, especially if coupled with other periods when deep muscle relaxation is practiced.

Sleep Apnea Syndrome

Sleep apnea literally means cessation of breathing during sleep. These apneas are usually repetitive and may last up to 60 seconds or even longer. Most sleep apnea syndromes result in excessive daytime sleepiness. (The disorder is discussed in detail later in this chapter.) Some patients, however, especially those who suffer from central sleep apneas, may complain exclusively about insomnia (Guilleminault and Dement, 1978).

Apnea syndromes are called central if they are due to failure of the neural control of breathing, or obstructive if they are due to obstruction of the airway. Clinically, the most commonly seen is a combination of initial central respiratory pause together with associated (and more dramatic) closure of the airway.

Central sleep apneas are difficult to diagnose without breath-monitoring equipment, because they usually do not manifest themselves in excessive snoring, gasping for air, or obesity, as do the upper airway sleep apneas. Also, such patients generally do not know about their sleep apneas, and those who complain about waking up with air hunger more likely suffer from some nocturnal panic attacks or night terrors. Bed partners may help by watching the patient's sleep, but the disorder may not be frequent enough to be seen while the partner is looking, and occasionally, there is merely a very shallow breathing rhythm, not complete cessation of breathing.

It is thought that central sleep apneas stem from a dysfunction in the lower respiratory centers or in the homeostatic mechanisms regulating blood gas levels. Treatment with medroxyprogesterone may increase respiratory drive and help in some cases (Strohl, Hensley, Saunders, et al, 1981). It is crucial not to prescribe hypnotics to such patients because those agents act as respiratory depressants, thus aggravating the problem. Indeed, one of the first clues (albeit not a very definite one) that central sleep apnea may be present is the patient's statement that many hypnotics have been tried in the past, but all have aggravated the insomnia.

Childhood-onset Insomnia

Previous chapters have discussed the complex neurological-neurochemical balances that decide whether at any given time the person is awake, asleep, or in REM. Given such a complex balance, it seems not surprising that these mechanisms may be dysfunctioning in some patients. If the balance tilts too much toward wakefulness, this neurological-neurochemical imbalance results in basic, primary insomnia.

Clinical experience has suggested that in most patients this problem has existed since birth, or at least since early childhood. Such patients often remember vividly being awake as young children when others slept. Not infrequently, childhood-onset insomnias are associated with attention-deficit disorders, other learning disabilities, mildly atypical EEGs of unknown significance even during adulthood, and other problems suggesting that all is not well neurologically (Hauri and Olmstead, 1980).

In general, patients with childhood-onset insomnia are extreme repressors, having learned throughout childhood and adolescence not to talk about their sleep difficulties for fear of rejection, ridicule, or being labeled "psychiatric." Those who finally are referred to sleep disorders centers seem to sleep much more poorly than patients with adult-onset insomnia (Hauri and Olmstead, 1980). Not only do they take longer to fall asleep and sleep less, they show ill-defined boundaries between sleep stages, and lack of spindles. Many of these patients are exquisitely sensitive to stimulants such as cola drinks, tea, or chocolate.

Clinically, we have found that very low doses of amitriptyline (10 to 50 mg at bedtime) often help such patients. Unlike the case with hypnotics, childhood-onset insomniacs do not seem to become habituated to the chronic use of amitriptyline.

Sleep-related Seizure Disorders

Some seizure disorders produce normal clinical EEGs during wakefulness but abnormal discharges at night. Depending on the type of seizure disorder, the transition between waking and sleeping (stage I), or delta sleep, or REM sleep might be particularly susceptible to epileptic discharges. Occasionally, such patients complain only about certain awakenings at night during which they feel extremely poorly. Sometimes these are postictal phenomena. In other patients, the sleep-related epilepsies, easier to diagnose, cause not only insomnia, but enuresis or night terrors.

Rarely does a standard somnogram sufficiently settle the question of nocturnal epilepsy, because for routine sleep staging only one or two EEG channels are recorded throughout the night. Rather, if nocturnal epilepsy is suspected, regular clinical EEG montages, possibly including nasopharyngeal leads and run at clinical speeds during the crucial times, seem necessary to document the problems. For such studies, routine sleep staging with eye and respiration monitors may not be necessary.

Nonrestorative Sleep

Some patients seem to sleep for adequate lengths of time, but feel worse in the morning than when they went to bed. Specifically, they complain about stiff, achy joints and muscles, excessive sensitivity to pain in the morning, and general malaise. These symptoms are not unlike those of rheumatoid arthritis, and in some patients, have led to the diagnosis of fibrositis (Moldofsky, Scarisbrick, England, 1975).

In the sleep EEG of many patients with nonrestorative sleep, one finds abundant, high-voltage alpha waves intruding into all NREM stages. Indeed, one can mimic the symptoms if one disturbs the sleep of normal volunteers by administering noise during NREM sleep. This either awakens the patients or brings them close to the arousal threshold, thus resulting in excessive alpha production (Moldofsky and Scarisbrick, 1976). A disturbance of REM sleep does not seem to lead to the symptoms.

It is interesting that nonrestorative sleep is much more difficult to produce in athletes. Even when athletes are awakened repeatedly from NREM sleep they do not develop the symptoms. This has led to the suggestion that increased exercise (e.g., swimming) might help such patients. Low doses of amitriptyline (10 to 50 mg at bedtime) seem to relieve the symptoms. Moldofsky and Lue (1980) have also shown that 100 mg of chlorpromazine abolish the alpha intrusions into sleep and make these people feel less stiff and achy in the morning, while L-tryptophan does not.

Idiopathic Insomnia

Having culled out all insomnias that are secondary to psychiatric and to medical dysfunctions, there remain those patients for whom poor sleep seems to be the only complaint. Usually this group contains 15 to 30 percent of all insomniacs, and the condition can be split into two main subsections.

Insomnia Complaints without Objective Findings

Everyone seems to know patients who claim that they "have not slept a wink," while those around them state that the patients slept all night, were unresponsive to disturbances, and possibly even snored loudly. In the sleep laboratory, such patients usually show totally normal sleep, at least insofar as this is recordable on the polygraph. Nevertheless, in the morning they claim again that they have slept very little.

Until recently, it was assumed that such patients were simply hypochondriacs, chronic complainers, or worse. While this may be true for some, there is now evidence that it may not be true for all of them. At the very least, many of these patients show daytime personality profiles and behavior that are not commensurate with a diagnosis of hypochondriasis (Piccione, Tallarigo, Zorick, et al, 1981). It would be difficult to postulate that these individuals are hypochondriacs about their sleep and normal concerning all other aspects of life. Also, there is evidence that these patients think more during bona fide sleep than do good sleepers (Hauri and Olmstead, 1983). Thus it may be that at least some of them suffer from an as yet undiscovered sleep disturbance that does not manifest itself in behavioral wakefulness or EEG sleep staging. Supporting this conclusion was the fact that, at least in our laboratory, many patients having an insomnia complaint without objective findings felt that they slept much better when given a hypnotic in a double-blind comparison with placebo. This was true even though the total amount of EEG-verified sleep had changed very little.

Persistent Psychophysiological Insomnia

Patients with persistent psychophysiological insomnia show chronically poor sleep, verifiable by behavioral observation or by EEG. There seems to be no readily apparent reason for this, either purely medical or obviously psychiatric.

It appears that two factors contribute to this condition: an organic (constitutional) predisposition toward poor sleep and a prolonged episode of severe stress. Neither factor alone is capable of triggering the insomnia; both must be present in the same individual.

The postulated organic factor may be understood as a predisposition toward poor sleep, possibly a mild form of childhood-onset insomnia. Patients with persistent psychophysiological insomnia often claim that before the stress they slept adequately, but not really well. Often, they state that throughout life they have suffered from one or two poor nights of sleep per month.

To understand the psychological components of psychophysiological insomnia, we can consider what happens to almost all of us during a period of excessive, prolonged stress. We sleep poorly because the stress increases activities in the arousal system, which is natural. As the stress and the poor sleep continue for weeks, we feel increasingly depleted and tired from lack of sleep. Obtaining a good night's sleep then becomes increasingly crucial because it becomes more and more difficult to function adequately without it. This development quite naturally leads to overconcern with sleep. One resolves to go to bed earlier and, consciously or unconsciously, tries harder and harder to sleep. This only leads to more and more wakefulness, because trying always causes arousal.

Conditioning is a second, almost unavoidable factor during a period of extreme insomnia due to stress. The more time one spends in bed frustrated and unable to sleep, the more the bed and its surroundings become associated with tension and frustration rather than with good sleep. After a while, just going into the bedroom, brushing teeth, and turning off the light become conditioned stimuli triggering frustration and arousal, while in the good sleeper the same stimuli may trigger relaxation and sleep.

Soon after the stress has disappeared, a basically good sleeper extinguishes the twin maladaptive factors of external conditioning and of trying too hard to sleep. Learning theory indicates that behavior that is never reinforced will soon extinguish. The patient with a constitutional sleep weakness, however, may never extinguish these maladaptive sleep-related habits because they are occasionally reinforced, which leads to chronically poor sleep for years and decades.

For the clinician, it seems important to distinguish which of the two factors discussed causes greater harm in a given individual. Patients who mainly try too hard to sleep often state that they can fall asleep whenever they would like to remain awake, for example, while watching television, in lectures, or while driving. As soon as they make a conscious decision to seek sleep, however, they become wide awake and tense, no matter where they try to sleep. On the other hand, those who suffer mainly from externally conditioned insomnia sleep best when the environment is different from their bedroom, for example, while camping, in motels, at friends' houses, on the floor, or in the sleep laboratory.

Making the distinction between the two learning factors that may cause psychophysiological insomnia is important because it leads to different treatments. The patient who tries too hard to sleep is encouraged to remain in bed trying to stay awake for as long as possible, reading a not-too-stimulating book, watching television, listening to radio programs, and the like. This procedure works only if the patient really tries to remain awake as long as possible and if a regular morning arousal time is strictly enforced no matter for how long the patient remained awake the night before. The patient with predominantly conditioned insomnia is asked not to read in bed, but to get out of bed and go into another room whenever sleep does not come easily. A procedure called stimulus control behavior therapy has been described elsewhere (Bootzin and Nicassio, 1978) and is quite efficient with such patients, but only if the therapist is well versed in behavior therapy and maintains close contact with the patients during the treatment. The list of rules for sleep hygiene suggests a useful additional regimen for such patients.

Patients with persistent psychophysiological insomnia will never become "champion" sleepers because they always carry their constitutional predisposition toward poor sleep. They can, however, often regain the type of sleep they had before the prolonged stress. In addition to the techniques described, many can benefit from relaxation training (Hauri, 1981; Borkovec and Weerts, 1976). It appears that those with persistent psychophysiological insomnia are extremely slow in learning relaxation techniques and they have to be very thoroughly trained before they are benefited. Also, some individuals seem neither anxious nor tense at sleep onset and still cannot sleep. For them, thorough relaxation training leads only to frustration and increased insomnia (Hauri, Percy, Hellekson, et al, 1982).

The occasional use of hypnotics is clearly indicated in psychophysiological insomnia. Initially, one tries to prevent maladaptive learning by prescribing almost daily hypnotics in patients undergoing severe stress if they have previously shown a predisposition toward poor sleep. In the later phases of the problem, hypnotics can be prescribed to be taken once or twice a week. This is done to allow patients some recovery sleep after a few poor nights; it also helps to alleviate feelings of panic when they fear that they may never sleep well again. Often, the knowledge that they can take a hypnotic tomorrow if sleep tonight is not adequate will ease the panic and allow the individuals to sleep without drugs.

There is no reason why only prolonged periods of stress may teach the twin maladaptive habits of trying too hard to sleep and external conditioning of insomnia. These habits can also be established if the original stress is medical—a prolonged episode of pain—or psychiatric—depression. In these cases, the behavioral techniques are used when the original stress condition is lifted, while the insomnia persists.

DISORDERS OF EXCESSIVE SOMNOLENCE

When sleep clinicians speak of excessive daytime somnolence (EDS), they mean an extreme propensity to fall asleep even after normal nights. Thus EDS is different from fatigue, malaise, hypothyroidism, or low-grade chronic depression. In the laboratory, the condition is assessed by having patients sleep for at least eight hours on the previous night, then having them take a 20-minute rest period every two hours during the following day (Richardson, Carskadon, Flagg et al, 1978). While normal subjects may fall asleep during one or two of these rest periods after a good night's sleep, those with EDS usually fall asleep in five minutes or less during each one. In the physician's office one cannot assess excessive sleepiness in this way. Rather, patients generally tell many anecdotes about how they actually fell asleep at the most inappropriate times: when driving, during an interview with the boss, while waiting on a customer, and so on.

While the symptoms may range from barely perceptible to severe, patients usually do not complain about EDS until the problem is quite disabling. People may deny such a problem as long as possible, since complaining about it is often interpreted as a sign of laziness. Ironically, once a diagnosis of EDS is made, almost all such patients turn out to have some medical organic disease. This situation is different from insomnia, in which most patients suffer from psychological or psychiatric disturbances. In EDS, the majority will have either sleep apnea or narcolepsy.

Sleep Apnea Syndrome

Sleep in patients with obstructive sleep apnea syndrome is usually characterized by loud, sonorous snoring or gasping for air alternating with periods of quiescence. Besides excessive daytime sleepiness, patients may also complain of very restless sleep, often associated with trancelike automatic behavior during the night, as well as night sweats, the need to take long, unrefreshing daytime naps, and headaches upon awakening. Many but not all of these patients are obese. Physical examination often reveals signs of right heart failure, that is, right ventricular enlargement and peripheral edema (Schroeder, Motta, and Guilleminault, 1978). Also, there are frequent and often serious cardiac arrhythmias ranging from premature ventricular contractions to prolonged sinus arrest (Tilkian, Motta, and Guilleminault, 1978; Tilkian, Guilleminault, Schroeder, et al, 1977). Hypertension is present in about 40 percent of cases.

Sleep clinicians distinguish three types of sleep apneas: upper airway obstructive apneas, in which respiratory movements are present but no air is exchanged because of an obstruction; central apneas, in which the upper airway remains open but no respiratory movements are made; and mixed apneas, that is, those that are first central but later become obstructive (Guilleminault and Dement, 1978). Many patients show all three types in any given night. Some have 500 and more apneas per night and spend up to 90 percent of their sleep not moving any air, while in other patients periods of apnea lasting from minutes to hours alternate with periods of normal sleep. Some have apneas only in REM sleep. Oxygen saturation is now routinely measured in these patients through ear oximetry. It often falls as low as 70 or 60 percent, if not lower.

There are many anatomical reasons for obstructive sleep apneas. In some patients, large tonsils, large uvulas, or other obstructions impede the flow of air. Others show retrognathia or micrognathia, placing the tongue too far to the back of the mouth where it can obstruct the airway during inspiration. Others have large, edematous soft palates (e.g., in hypothyroidism) or congenitally small airways. Fat deposits around the airway may also compromise air flow during sleep (Coccagna, Cirignotta, and Lugaresi, 1978; Orr, Males, and Imes, 1981; Harper and Sauerland, 1978). During sleep, the musculature around the upper airway relaxes and the lumen naturally gets much smaller. In other cases, a genetic component seems to be present. In most patients, however, there is no readily assessable etiology. Sleep apneas are about 60 times more frequent in men than in premenopausal women. The incidence seems to increase among women after menopause, but in varying severity and degree in different studies.

Treatment depends on the severity of the disease. How sleepy is the person during the day? What is the cardiac status, the level of oxygen desaturation reached at night, and so forth? In mild cases, relief may be found if the patients sleep in a chair. If the problem is not urgent, weight loss may be tried first. Obstructions might be surgically corrected and hypothyroidism treated to help shrink the soft palate. Protriptyline has helped in some patients who experienced fewer than 30 apneas per hour (Conway, Zorick, Piccione, et al, 1982). A procedure called uvulo-palato-pharyngoplasty (UPP) has shown surprisingly beneficial results in many patients (Fujita, Zorick, Conway, et al, 1980). In this operation, the skin and musculature around the upper airway are tightened and fat deposits removed. Finally, in severe cases, especially when cardiac status is alarming, a permanent tracheostomy is implanted, open during the night for breathing, closed during the day for normal talking.

While the incidence of sleep apnea increases with age (Ancoli-Israel, Kripke, Mason, et al, 1981), no age group is spared. Many cases of sudden infant death syndrome (SIDS) apparently can be traced to sleep apneas in the 3- to 6-month-old. Some cases of supposed mental retardation in children have been traced to sleep apnea, with gratifying results once the problem is surgically corrected.

Estimates about the incidence of sleep apnea syndromes have been continuously revised upward during the last decade. In many sleep disorders centers, these are now the most frequently seen conditions. It seems hard to believe that only 15 years ago very few researchers and clinicians were even aware that they existed.

Narcolepsy

The disorder of narcolepsy was described more than 100 years ago as a neurological condition occurring in dogs and other mammals. The problem could not be understood, however, until some of the sleep mechanisms, such as the REM/NREM cycle, had been discovered (Dement, Carskadon, Guilleminault, and Zarcone, 1976).

Narcolepsy is now best conceptualized as an imbalance between the wake/NREM/REM systems. Wakefulness seems weak, easily overpowered by an excessively strong REM system. This REM system is often triggered by emotions such as laughter or anger (Karacan, Moore, and Williams, 1979). It can intrude into wakefulness either partially or totally, giving rise to the narcoleptic tetrad:

1.   Excessive daytime sleepiness: Although narcoleptics seem to be chronically tired and sleep very poorly at night, they do seem to get some short-lived benefit from frequent, short, daytime naps. Such naps should be encouraged where possible.

2.   Cataplexy: Sometimes, when only the muscle paralysis part of REM sleep is triggered, the narcoleptic remains awake but paralyzed. This paralysis can range from a very transient weakness in the patient's knees or a slight jaw dropping during excitement to a total collapse and falling helplessly to the floor.
3.   Sleep paralysis: This is a type of cataplexy that occurs either at sleep onset or immediately after awakening. Only sleep-onset paralysis seems indicative of narcolepsy, however. Transient paralysis when awakening from REM sleep is much more widespread and more benign, albeit frightening. It is rarely associated with narcolepsy.
4.   Hypnagogic hallucinations: REM dreaming may occur before the narcoleptic loses consciousness at sleep onset. This means that some patients actually see the vivid images of dreaming even though they are still in contact with a waking consciousness.

Not every narcoleptic suffers from all four symptoms of the narcoleptic tetrad. When cataplexy, sleep-onset paralysis, or hypnagogic hallucinations coexist with excessive daytime sleepiness, it is diagnostic of narcolepsy. In addition, other symptoms may occur, such as automatic behavior that may resemble psychomotor seizures or amnesia for short periods during the day. These episodes are apparently related to the narcoleptic's decreased arousal levels. The patient's behavior during these episodes seems appropriate for routine activities (e.g., driving), but recall is impaired, reaction time may be slowed, and judgment is clouded.

In the laboratory, narcoleptics may show a sleep-onset REM period, that is, they may slip from wakefulness directly into REM sleep. Depending on the severity of the condition, this might happen every night or not even once a week. Therefore an incidence of falling asleep without going through a REM period does not rule out narcolepsy. The situation is further confused by the fact that even some non-narcoleptics may have sleep-onset REM periods under certain conditions, for example, when withdrawn from REM-suppressant agents such as amphetamines or alcohol, when falling asleep at highly unusual hours such as in a morning nap, or when endogenously depressed.

Narcolepsy usually starts in the second or third decade of life. Initially, only one symptom of the tetrad may be present, and problems may gradually increase. Once the disorder is fully established, it seems to remain relatively stable throughout the rest of the patient's life (Kales, Cadieux, Soldatos, et al, 1982).

The incidence of narcolepsy is estimated at about 4 per 10,000 equally distributed between males and females. Relatives of narcoleptics have more than a 60-fold higher risk of developing the condition. Thus there is clearly a genetic component.

While narcolepsy is a physiological disease, it takes a heavy psychological toll (Kales, Soldatos, Bixler, et al, 1982). Narcoleptics are often considered lazy because of frequent napping. Those whose condition is severe may refuse to leave their homes for fear of having cataplectic attacks in public. Some misinterpret their hypnagogic hallucinations as manifestations of psychosis. To receive some of the emotional support that they need, narcoleptics may be referred to a self-help group: The American Narcolepsy Association (P.O. Box 5846, Stanford, CA 94305).

So far, there is no truly adequate treatment for everybody with narcolepsy. One tries to bolster wakefulness by stimulant drugs, ranging from coffee through pemoline and methylphenidate to amphetamines (Zarcone, 1973; Schmidt, Clark, and Hyman, 1977; Scrima, 1982; Campbell, 1981). Depending on the severity of the disease, some narcoleptics need stimulants only occasionally, such as before a long car drive. Others may need it daily. The lowest possible stimulant dose is selected to delay habituation, and narcoleptics are encouraged to take at least one or two naps per day. Cataplexy responds to REM suppressant medication, either imipramine or protriptyline. Recently, some researchers have suggested treatment with γ-hydroxybutyrate (Mamelak and Webster, 1981).

Other Disorders of Excessive Somnolence

While over two-thirds of all patients with serious excessive somnolence seem to have either sleep apnea or narcolepsy, there are several other disorders that are relatively difficult to diagnose (see Table 5.1). Some patients may have idiopathic CNS hypersomnolence, a little-understood condition that is possibly related to neurochemical imbalances (Van den Hoed, Kraemer, Guilleminault, et al, 1981). Others may suffer from nocturnal myoclonus or other types of insomnia that cause excessive sleepiness during the day. Depression, especially in young adults, may occasionally lead to hypersomnolence rather than to insomnia (Hawkins, Taub, Van de Castle, et al, 1977). Others may simply not get enough sleep. Finally, periodic hypersomnolence may be related to menses (Billiard, Guilleminault, and Dement, 1975), or it may indicate the rare Kleine-Levin syndrome (Orlosky, 1982). Because all of these forms of hypersomnolence seem rather rare and complex, their treatment is best left to the specialist.

DISORDERS OF THE SLEEP-WAKE SCHEDULE

As discussed earlier, sleep is embedded in the circadian rhythm, part of the diurnal ebb and flow that includes all organic functioning and involves metabolism, body temperature, and hormone secretion, as well as sleep. Not only is it easier to sleep at certain clock times, but sleep itself, especially the time of awakening, may act as a powerful zeitgeber (time clue). This means that regular arousal times can help to synchronize circadian rhythms and associate them with the exact clock time that is imposed on us by the rotation of our planet.

A detailed discussion of circadian rhythms, their interactions, and their anatomical, neurochemical, and physiological concomitants is beyond the limits of this chapter. Because many abnormalities that are based on this rhythm can masquerade as sleep disturbances, they are briefly mentioned here.

Frequently Changing Sleep-Wake Schedule

Basically, humans can learn to sleep well during any time of the day or night, as long as that time is held rigidly consistent over a few weeks. When the time of sleeping changes frequently, as in rotating shift work or when shiftworkers sleep during the night on their days off but during the day when working, circadian rhythms can become disorganized. Individuals then may develop not only sleep difficulties, but mood changes and cognitive difficulties, even organic problems such as peptic ulcers. There is a wide variability in adaptability to shift work. While some thrive on a varied schedule all their lives, others have difficulties reestablishing a consolidated sleep period even after they have ceased shift work (Aschoff, Hoffman, Pohl, 1975; Halberg, 1976).

Delayed and Advanced Sleep Phase Syndrome

Some people, especially younger ones, habitually go to sleep in the early morning hours and then sleep until afternoon. Older persons often show the opposite: going to bed very early, then awaking long before morning. Such individuals may have difficulties returning to more conventional sleep times when it becomes necessary to do so (Weitzman, 1981).

It seems unclear whether the delayed sleep syndrome typical of young adulthood and the advanced sleep syndrome typical of old age are basically social phenomena, or whether organic components play the key role. When normalization is desired, it has been demonstrated that "going with the rhythm" is more effective than fighting it. Thus in a treatment called chronotherapy, patients with delayed sleep syndromes are asked to delay their sleep even further if they want to sleep during conventional hours (Czeisler, Richardson, Coleman, 1981). For example, a young adult habitually going to bed at 5 AM might delay sleep three hours each day. Thus he would go to bed at 8 AM on the first day, 11 AM on the second, and so on, until he has reached a conventionally acceptable evening bedtime. At that time, it becomes crucial to stabilize the rhythm by rigidly adhering to a conventional morning arousal time.

Non-24-Hour Sleep-Wake Syndrome

While most humans seem to have an innate circadian rhythm of somewhere around 25 hours, it appears that in some of us this internal rhythm is much longer, possibly 30 to 40 hours. Such people go to bed progressively later each night. Their problem often seems periodic. During some time periods, when their internal rhythms coincide with society's, they sleep and work well. During other times, however, when their rhythms are opposite to those of society, they obtain very little sleep at night and have extreme difficulties functioning during the day and keeping normal jobs.

To diagnose a non-24-hour sleep-wake syndrome, patients record their sleep and arousal times for at least three weeks. They rarely are aware that they have a slowed rhythm, but complain only about periodic insomnia or periodic excessive sleepiness. While some individuals with this problem can learn to conform to society's demands by sheer willpower, others select more independent jobs such as free-lance work. Recently, some have had success with monthly chronotherapy, rotating around the clock for about one week, then holding bedtime rigidly constant for about three weeks.

Irregular Sleep-Wake Patterns

Although we may bemoan it daily, the regular schedule imposed on most of us by our work helps to keep an adequate 24-hour rhythm. There are situations where such rhythms are lost, such as during chronic sickness, when one lies in bed dozing day and night, or for persons with few social ties and independent jobs that can be carried out any time, day or night (Kokkoris, Weitzman, Pollack, et al, 1978; Miles, Raynal, and Wilson, 1977). Not only does the circadian rhythm disassociate itself from the usual day-night rhythm in these instances, but different aspects of the rhythm may start to take on different lengths. Core body temperature, for example, may follow a 24-hour rhythm, while sleep-wake cycle may follow a 33-hour rhythm. Often, such patients then complain that they can only sleep in short naps and that they are always sleepy, but never sleeping well.

Treatment of irregular patterns consists in gradually reestablishing a circadian rhythm. Initially, there is only a short time during each day when the patient is forced to remain awake, for example, from noon until 3 PM. Gradually that time is expanded, until the regular 16 to 18 hours of continuous wakefulness are reached. It is rarely possible for patients themselves to regain a lost circadian rhythm; more often, external help is needed initially to enforce the rhythm.

A similar problem may occur in older persons after retirement. Having lost the external impetus to be up and at work each day at a certain time, they may first luxuriate in the feeling of freedom to sleep and wake whenever they please. Later, this may turn against them as their rhythms desynchronize.

PARASOMNIAS

Disturbances that occur during sleep or during partial arousals from sleep are called parasomnias. Some are tied to specific sleep stages; others are not. For example, it is very difficult to awaken from delta sleep. When disturbed in that type of sleep, it takes most of us a few seconds to become oriented. Others, especially children whose delta sleep is even deeper, not only have difficulties becoming oriented when disturbed in delta sleep, they cannot do so at all. They then enter a "confusional" state, half asleep and half awake, in which certain parasomnias such as night terrors and somnambulism may occur.

Sleep-related Epileptic Seizures

Although sleep epilepsy seems relatively rare, the clinician must always keep in mind that many parasomnias such as sleepwalking, night terrors, and enuresis may be triggered by sleep-related epileptic phenomena, especially temporal lobe problems. In many of these cases, the daytime clinical EEG is totally normal (Kooi, Tucker and Marshall, 1978; Riley, 1983). Sometimes, the abnormal discharges cannot be seen even in the sleeping clinical EEG except when nasopharyngeal or sphenoidal leads are used. Also, while some of these seizure problems manifest themselves almost as soon as the patient falls asleep, others need a few hours of sleep before the abnormal spikes and waves appear. Thus specialized all-night EEGs may be necessary to rule out sleep-related seizures. To complicate matters, many clinically normal individuals may show atypical EEG waves while asleep, such as 6- and 14-Hz positive spikes, 6-Hz spike and wave complexes, or small sharp spikes. These events are insufficient to diagnose epilepsy. Often, concomitant sleep EEG and behavioral observations are necessary to decide on a final diagnosis.

The Distinction between Night Terrors and
Dream Anxiety Attacks

Night terrors are delta sleep phenomena. Patients, especially children, usually start their night terrors with a blood-curdling scream about one-half to one hour after sleep onset. They then show many autonomic signs of extreme panic, such as a doubling or tripling of the heart rate, sweating, respiratory distress, or pupil dilation. Usually, they are very hard to arouse during their terrors. Most often they calm down by themselves within a few minutes and then return to sleep. On the rare occasions when they come to full consciousness, they may relate one or two pieces of very short, frightening imagery such as "the walls are tumbling down," "there is a bull in my room," or "I could not catch my breath" (Fisher, Kahn, Edwards, 1973; Kales, Soldatos, Caldwell, et al, 1980). For most there is total amnesia for the terrors in the morning, and other family members seem more concerned about the episodes than the sleeper.

Dream anxiety attacks arise from REM sleep and usually occur during the later parts of the night, when dreams are longer, more vivid, and emotional. Although there may be some moaning and thrashing around during the dream anxiety attack, usually there are neither the screams nor the other signs of extreme autonomic arousal that are found in night terrors. Those suffering from dream anxiety attacks can usually relate fairly elaborate, frightening dream content (Kramer, 1979). Frequently, their dreams are repetitive, the same content disturbing the dreamer night after night.

Night terrors are distinguished easily from dream anxiety attacks by asking two questions: At what time of the night does the disturbance occur, and how much can the dreamer remember? Making the distinction is important in the case of children. It appears that night terrors in children are basically biological phenomena that do not indicate psychiatric distress (Kales, Soldatos, Caldwell, 1980). Psychotherapy is not required. This is true even though night terrors often occur more frequently when the child is under stress. Dream anxiety attacks usually need some psychological resolution, that is, psychotherapy.

In adults, the distinction between night terrors and dream anxiety attacks becomes less crucial because those suffering from either problem may require psychotherapy. In addition, a new form of "nightmare" appears in adults. Some patients, especially those suffering from posttraumatic stress disorders and from the initial phases of psychosis, may experience frightening imagery during the transition phase between wakefulness and sleep (i.e., during stage I). Some spend long hours in this transition phase throughout the night.

Benzodiazepines, especially diazepam, appear to abolish both night terrors and dream anxiety attacks. While one will not chronically prescribe this medication for children just because of nightmares, an occasional low dose of diazepam may be indicated for a night when such nightmares might be embarrassing, such as when spending the night with friends.

Somnambulism

Sleepwalking usually starts with a burst of high-voltage delta waves, then the EEG flattens somewhat, and the person starts to move about. As with night terrors, episodes of somnambulism are carried out in a confusional state, partly awake, partly asleep. The patient usually is aware enough to perform relatively simple behaviors such as avoiding furniture, opening doors, even starting a car, but reactions are dull and judgment is clouded. For example, people have walked out of windows thinking they were doors, urinated in a corner of a room thinking that they are in the bathroom, or attacked family members, mistaking them for enemies. Somnambulists are usually uncommunicative during the episodes, and most often, spontaneously either return to bed or curl up and sleep somewhere else. As with those suffering from night terrors, somnambulists are usually difficult to bring to full consciousness during the events. In general, they are totally amnesic for the episodes the next morning.

Sleepwalking in children is generally benign. It commonly starts before the age of 10 and stops by age 15. Episodes are usually infrequent and can sometimes be triggered by disturbing the child during delta sleep, for example, by placing the child gently on his feet. There is no evidence that these children are more psychologically disturbed than those who do not sleepwalk (Kales, Soldatos, Caldwell, 1980b).

Somnambulism in adults is more serious. If it occurs frequently, if often indicates excessive tension or stress, if not outright psychopathology. Once nocturnal epilepsy and drug reactions are ruled out, adult somnambulists may need psychotherapy.

Occasionally, somnambulism is secondary to medication such as hypnotics (Huapaya, 1979) or combined lithium-neuroleptic treatment (Charney, Kales, Soldatos, 1979). The deeper delta sleep is and the more there is of it during a given night, the more likely somnambulism becomes. Thus patients prone to this problem should avoid sleep deprivation or agents that produce increased delta sleep, such as alcohol.

Somnambulism must be differentiated from organic brain syndrome with confusion (the so-called sundowner's syndrome) in older patients, and from hysteric fugues, which allow much more complex and purposeful behavior than somnambulism. Also, some malingering may be carried out under the guise of somnambulism, such as raiding the refrigerator at night without having to accept blame.

Treatment to date is unsatisfactory. Some have claimed success with diazepam (Reid and Gutnik, 1980), imipramine, amphetamine, and anticonvulsants (Pedley and Guilleminault, 1977). Some patients respond to behavior therapy or hypnosis (Reid, Ahmed, and Levie, 1981). In general, however, the main concern is for the patients' safety. Frequent somnambulists should sleep on the ground floor and not have nighttime access to dangerous objects such as knives, guns, and car keys. Their spouses might have to learn some hand-holds to free themselves and restrain the somnambulist should that ever become necessary.

Sleep-related Enuresis

Our culture puts a premium on early maturation because this is thought to indicate high intelligence. Thus many parents exaggerate the early time that their offspring first have dry nights, or they deny bedwetting in their older children. This has led to exaggerated expectations. Indeed, frequent bed-wetting is still found in about 10 percent of girls and 15 percent of boys at age 5 years (Anders, 1976).

Primary enuresis is the term used to indicate that nocturnal toilet train-ing has never been accomplished. Secondary enuresis indicates bedwetting that recurs or relapses after a few weeks or months of dryness. The latter is more likely to be psychogenic, while the former may be symptomatic of organic etiology. Most enuresis is nonorganic, a self-limited phenomenon apparently based on delayed maturation (Shaffer, 1977). Indeed, after a careful study of 40 severely enuretic boys, Mikkelsen et al (1980) suggested that detailed urological investigations should not be carried out in enuretic children unless prior evidence by history suggests organic pathology. At least, if the parents have a history of enuresis that later normalized spon-taneously, it seems likely that the same will happen in their children at about the same age.

Little has been added to the treatment of enuresis during the last few years. Behavioral techniques seem quite successful, such as stars for dry nights or the bell-and-blanket technique, as long as the therapist or parent is reasonably sensitive to the child's needs. Imipramine (10 to 75 mg at bedtime) may abolish enuresis (Mikkelson et al, 1980), at least for the du-ration of treatment. While one might not consider chronic treatment with this drug in children, it may seem indicated for the occasional nights when bedwetting must not occur, such as when the child spends nights with friends. The appropriate dosage must first be carefully titrated to each child's needs.

Other Parasomnias

As Table 5.1 indicates, there is a large list of additional parasomnias. Be-cause they are rare, each is mentioned only briefly here, and the physician is referred to the appropriate literature.

Sleep-related bruxism occurs in two forms. One is diurnal bruxism—tooth grinding during both night and day. This is possibly related to stress and seems treatable by biofeedback. The other is nocturnal bruxism—tooth grinding only during sleep and apparently not related to stress (Glaros, 1981). Diurnal bruxism seems amenable to biofeedback therapy; nocturnal bruxism is often treated with a toothguard.

Sleep-related head banging or head-and-body rocking often seems to be a comfort habit, similar to thumb sucking (Baldy-Moulinier, Levy, and Passouant, 1970).

In some patients, familial sleep paralysis occurs frequently when awakening from REM sleep. It seems to be benign and rarely develops into full-blown narcolepsy (Hishikawa, 1976).

Sleep-related cluster headaches and chronic paroxysmal hemicrania seem to be of vascular origin and associated with REM sleep (Kayed, Godtlibsen, and Sjaastad, 1978).

Most sleep-related cardiovascular symptoms relate to prolonged recumbence rather than sleep. The low systemic blood pressure typical for delta sleep and the elevated and highly variable blood pressure associated with REM sleep may also be involved (Rosenblatt, Hartmann, and Zwilling, 1978).

Acid clearing seems delayed during sleep, and patients predisposed to sleep-related gastroesophageal reflux may awaken from sleep either with heartburn or with a sour taste in the mouth. If untreated, complications such as esophageal stricture or aspiration pneumonia may develop (Orr, Hall, Stahl et al, 1976).

CONCLUSION

This chapter summarizes what most physicians need to know to deal with sleep disorders. It is a fascinating field, where a skillful combination of medical, pharmacological, and behavioral approaches often can achieve success, if they are carefully blended. As implied, most diagnoses and treatments initially lie within the grasp of the general practitioner, with the possible exception of diagnosing difficult cases of excessive daytime sleepiness. In those cases prompt referral to a sleep disorders specialist seems indicated because one may be dealing with a possibly life-threatening situation.

Should other sleep disorders such as insomnia or parasomnias remain serious and relentless even after the best efforts of the general physician have been spent, referral to a sleep disorders specialist might then be considered. While such referrals are not cheap, neither is the prolonged, chronic treatment of a misdiagnosed sleep disorder, not only in terms of money, but in terms of stresses caused by these problems to self, family, and society.

REFERENCES

Ancoli-Israel S, Kripke DF, Mason W, et al. Sleep apnea and nocturnal myoclonus in a senior population. Sleep 1981;4:349–58.

Anders TF. What we know about sleep disorders in children. Med Times 1976;104:75–80.

Aschoff J, Hoffman K, Pohl H. Reentrainment of circadian rhythms after phase-shifts of the zeitgeber. Chronobiologia 1975;2:23–78.

Association of Sleep Disorders Centers. Diagnostic classification of sleep and arousal disorders. 1st ed. Prepared by the Sleep Disorders Classification Committee, Roffwarg HP, Chairman. Sleep 1979;2(1):1–137.

Baekeland F, Lasky R. Exercise and sleep patterns in college athletes. Percept Motor Skills 1966;23:1203–7.

Baldy-Moulinier M, Levy M, Passouant P. A study of jactatio capitis during night sleep. Electroencephalogr Clin Neurophysiol 1970;28:87.

Billiard M, Guilleminault WC, Dement WC. A menstruation-linked periodic hypersomnia. Neurology (Minneap) 1975;25:436–43.

Bootzin RR, Nicassio PN. Behavioral treatments for insomnia. In: Hersen M, Eisler R, Miller P, eds. Progress in behavior modification. New York: Academic Press, 1978.

Borkovec TD, Lane TW, VanOot PH. Phenomenology of sleep among insomniacs and good sleepers: wakefulness experience when cortically asleep. J Abnorm Psychol 1981;90(6):607–9.

Borkovec TD, Weerts TD. Effects of progressive relaxation on sleep disturbance: an electroencephalographic evaluation. Psychosom Med 1976;38:173–80.

Brezinova V, Oswald I. Sleep after a bedtime beverage. Br Med J 1972;2:431–33.

Campbell RK. The treatment of narcolepsy and cataplexy. Drug Intel Clin Pharm 1981;15:257–62.

Charney DS, Kales A, Soldatos CR. Somnambulistic-like episodes secondary to combined lithium-neuroleptic treatment. Br J Psychiatry 1979;135:418–24.

Coccagna G, Cirignotta F, Lugaresi E. The bird-like face syndrome (acquired micrognathia, hypersomnia, and sleep apnea). In: Guilleminault WC, Dement WC, eds. Sleep apnea syndromes. New York: Alan R. Liss, 1978:259–72.

Coleman RM. Periodic movement in sleep (nocturnal myoclonus) and restless legs syndrome. In: Guilleminault WC, ed. Sleeping and waking disorders: indications and techniques. Menlo Park, Calif.: Addison-Wesley, 1982:265–96.

Conway WA, Zorick F, Piccione P, Roth T. Protriptyline in the treatment of sleep apnea. Thorax 1982;37:49–53.

Coursey RD, Frankel BL. Novelty-seeking, fantasy, and sensitization in chronic insomniacs. Percept Motor Skills 1977;44:795–98.

Czeisler CA, Richardson GS, Coleman RM. Chronotherapy: resetting the circadian clocks of patients with delayed sleep phase insomnia. Sleep 1981;4:1–21.

Dement WC, Carskadon MA, Guilleminault WC, Zarcone VP. Narcolepsy: diagnosis and treatment. Primary Care 1976;3(3):609–23.

Evans FJ, Cook MR, Cohen HD. Appetitive and replacement naps: EEG and behavior. Science 1977;197:687–89.

Fisher C, Kahn E, Edwards A. A psychophysiological study of nightmares and night terrors: the suppression of stage IV night terrors with diazepam. Arch Gen Psychiatry 1973;28:252–59.

Frankel BL, Patten BM, Gillin JC. Restless legs syndrome. Sleep-electroencephalographic and neurologic findings. JAMA 1974;230:1302–3.

Fujita S, Zorick F, Conway W, et al. Uvulo-palato-pharyngoplasty: a new surgical treatment for upper airway sleep apnea. In: Chase MH, Stern WC, Walter PL, eds. Sleep research. Los Angeles: Brain Information Service/Brain Research Institute, UCLA, 1980;9:197 (abstract).

Glaros AG. Incidence of diurnal and nocturnal bruxism. Prosthet Dent 1981;45:545–49.

Globus G, Friedmann J, Cohen H, et al. The effects of aircraft noise on sleep electrophysiology as recorded in the home. In: Ward WD, ed. Proceedings of the International Congress on Noise as a Public Health Problem. Washington, D.C.: U.S. Environmental Protection Agency, 1974:587–91.

Griffin SJ, Trinder J. Physical fitness, exercise, and human sleep. Soc Psychophysiol Res 1978;15(5):447–50.

Guilleminault WC, Dement WC. Sleep apnea syndromes and related sleep disorders. In: Williams RL, Karacan I, eds. Sleep disorders: diagnosis and treatment. New York: John Wiley & Sons, 1978:9–28.

Halberg F. Some aspects of chronobiology relating to the optiminization of shift work. In: Rentos RG, Shepard RD, eds. Shift work and health: a symposium. U.S. Department of Health, Education and Welfare, National Institute for Occupational Safety and Health, Office of Extramural Activities. Washington, D.C.: The Department, 1976:13–47.

Harper RM, Sauerland EK. The role of the tongue in sleep apnea. In: Guilleminault WC, Dement WC, eds. Sleep apnea syndromes. New York: Alan R. Liss, 1978:219–34.

Hauri P. Treating psychophysiologic insomnia with biofeedback. Arch Gen Psychiatry 1981;38:752–58.

Hauri P. The sleep disorders: current concepts. Kalamazoo, Mich.: Upjohn Scope Publications, 1982:14.

Hauri P, Olmstead E. Childhood-onset insomnia. Sleep 1980;3:59–65.

Hauri P, Olmstead E. What is the moment of sleep onset for insomniacs? Sleep 1983;6(1):10–15.

Hauri PJ, Percy L, Hellekson C, et al. The treatment of psychophysiologic insomnia with biofeedback: a replication study. Biofeedback and Sleep Regulation 1982;7:223–35.

Hawkins DR, Taub JM, Van de Castle RL, et al. Sleep stage patterns associated with depression in young adult patients. In: Koella WP, Levin P, eds. Sleep nineteen seventy-six. Memory, environment, epilepsy, sleep staging. Basel: S. Karger, 1977:424–27.

Hishikawa Y. Sleep paralysis. In: Guilleminault WC, Dement WC, Passouant P, eds. Advances in sleep research. Narcolepsy. Proceedings of the first international symposium on narcolepsy, Montpellier, France, July 1975. New York: Spectrum, 1976:97–124.

Huapaya LVM. Seven cases of somnambulism induced by drugs. Am J Psychiatry 1979;136:985–86.

Jacobs BL, McGinty DJ. Effects of food deprivation on sleep and wakefulness in the rat. Exp Neurol 1971;30:212–22.

Johnson LC. Psychological and physiological changes following total sleep deprivation. In: Kales AA, ed. Sleep physiology and pathology. Philadelphia: JB Lippincott, 1969:206–220.

Johnson LC. Are stages of sleep related to waking behavior? Am Sci 1973;61:326–38.

Johnson LC, Burdick JA, Smith J. Sleep during alcohol intake and withdrawal in the chronic alcoholic. Arch Gen Psychiatry 1970;22:406–18.

Kales A, Bixler EO, Soldatos CR, et al. Biopsychobehavioral correlates of insomnia. I. Role of sleep apnea and nocturnal myoclonus. Psychosomatics 1982;23:589–600.

Kales A, Cadieux RJ, Soldatos CR, et al. Narcolepsy-cataplexy. I. Clinical and electrophysiologic characteristics. Arch Neurol 1982;39:164–68.

Kales A, Soldatos CR, Bixler EO, et al. Narcolepsy-cataplexy. II. Psychosocial consequences and associated psychopathology. Arch Neurol 1982;39:169–71.

Kales A, Soldatos CR, Caldwell AB, et al. Nightmares: clinical characteristics and personality patterns. Am J Psychiatry 1980a;137:1197–1201.

Kales A, Soldatos CR, Caldwell AB, et al. Somnambulism. Arch Gen Psychiatry 1980b;37:1406–10.

Kales A, Tan TL, Kollar EJ, et al. Sleep patterns following 205 hours of sleep deprivation. Psychosom Med 1970;32:189–200.

Karacan I, Moore CA, Williams RL. The narcoleptic syndrome. Psychiatr Ann 1979;9(7):377–81.

Karacan I, Thornby JI, Anch AM, et al. Dose-related sleep disturbances induced by coffee and caffeine. Clin Pharmacol Ther 1976;20:682–89.

Kayed K, Godtlibsen OB, Sjaastad O. Chronic paroxysmal hemicrania. IV. REM sleep-locked nocturnal headache attacks. Sleep 1978;1:91–95.

Kokkoris CP, Weitzman ED, Pollak CP, et al. Long-term ambulatory temperature monitoring in a subject with a hypernychthemeral sleep-wake cycle disturbance. Sleep 1978;1:177–90.

Kooi KA, Tucker RP, Marshall RE. Fundamentals of electroencephalography. 2nd ed. New York: Harper & Row, 1978.

Kramer M. Dream disturbances. Psychiatr Annu 1979;366–76.

Lutz EG. Restless legs, anxiety and caffeinism. J Clin Psychiatry 1978;39:693–98.

Mamelak M, Webster P. Treatment of narcolepsy and sleep apnea with gamma-hydroxybutyrate: a clinical and polysomnographic case study. Sleep 1981;4:105–11.

Meddis R, Pearson AJD, Langford G. An extreme case of healthy insomnia. Electroencephalogr Clin Neurophysiol 1973;35:213–14.

Mikkelsen EJ, Rapoport JL, Nee I. Childhood enuresis. I. Sleep patterns and psychopathology. Arch Gen Psychiatry 1980;37:1139–44.

Miles LEM, Raynal DM, Wilson MA. Blind man living in normal society has circadian rhythms of 24.9 hours. Science 1977;198:421–23.

Moldofsky H, Lue FA. The relationship of alpha and delta EEG frequencies to pain and mood in fibrositis patients treated with chlorpromazine and L-tryptophan. Electroencephalogr Clin Neurophysiol 1980;50:71–80.

Moldofsky H, Scarisbrick P. Induction of neurasthenic musculoskeletal pain syndrome by selective sleep stage deprivation. Psychosom Med 1976;38:35–44.

Moldofsky H, Scarisbrick P, England R, et al. Musculoskeletal symptoms and non-REM sleep disturbance in patients with fibrositis syndrome and healthy subjects. Psychosom Med 1975;37:341–51.

Morgan BB. Effects of continuous work and sleep loss in the reduction and recovery of work efficiency. Am Indust Hyg Assoc J 1974:13–20.

Mullaney DJ, Johnson LC, Naitoh P, et al. Sleep during and after gradual sleep reduction. Psychophysiology 1977;14:237–44.

Myrsten AL, Elgerot A, Edgren B. Effects of abstinence from tobacco smoking on physiological and psychological arousal levels in habitual smokers. Psychosom Med 1977;39:25–38.

Orlosky MJ. The Kleine-Levin syndrome: a review. Psychosomatics 1982;23(6):609–21.

Orr WC, Hall WH, Stahl ML. Sleep patterns and gastric acid secretion in duodenal ulcer disease. Arch Intern Med 1976;136:655–60.

Orr WC, Males JL, Imes NK. Myxedema and obstructive sleep apnea. Am J Med 1981;70:1061–66.

Otto E. Physiological analysis of sleep disturbances induced by noise and increased room temperature. In: Koella WP, Levin P, eds. Sleep, first European congress on sleep research, Basel, Switzerland, October 3–6, 1972. Basel: S. Karger, 1973:414–18.

Pasnau RO, Naitoh P, Stier S, Kollar EJ. The psychological effects of 205 hours of sleep deprivation. Arch Gen Psychiatry 1968;18:496–505.

Pedley TA, Guilleminault WC. Episodic nocturnal wanderings responsive to anticonvulsant drug therapy. Ann Neurol 1977;2:30–35.

Piccione P, Tallarigo R, Zorick F, et al. Personality differences between insomniac and non-insomniac psychiatry outpatients. J Clin Psychiatry 1981;42(7):261–63.

Reid WH, Ahmed I, Levie CA. Treatment of sleep-walking: a controlled study. Am J Psychother 1981;85:27–37.

Reid WH, Gutnik BD. Case report: treatment of intractable sleepwalking. Psychiatr J Univ Ottawa 1980;5:86–88.

Richardson GS, Carskadon MA, Flagg W. Excessive daytime sleepiness in man: multiple sleep latency measurements in narcoleptic and control subjects. Electroencephalogr Clin Neurophysiol 1978;45:621–27.

Riley TL. Electroencephalography in diagnosis and management of epilepsy. In: Brown T, Feldman R, eds. Epilepsy. Boston: Little, Brown, 1983:23–40.

Rosenblatt G, Hartmann E, Zwilling GR. Cardiac irritability during sleep and dreaming. J Psychosom Res 1978;17:129–34.

Schmidt HS, Clark RW, Hyman PR. Protriptyline: an effective agent in the treatment of the narcolepsy-cataplexy syndrome and hypersomnia. Am J Psychiatry 1977;84:183–85.

Schmidt-Kessen W, Kendel K. Einfluss der Raumtemperatur auf den Nachtschlaf. Res Exp Med (Berlin) 1973;160:220–33.

Schroeder JS, Motta J, Guilleminault WC. Hemodynamic studies in sleep apnea. In: Guilleminault WC, Dement WC, eds. Sleep apnea syndromes. New York: Alan R. Liss, 1978:177–95.

Scrima L. Letter to the editor. Sleep 1982;5(1):110.

Shaffer D. Enuresis. In: Rutter M, Hersov C, eds. Child psychiatry: modern approaches. London: Blackwell Scientific Publications, 1977:581–612.

Soldatos CR, Kales JD, Scharf MB. Cigarette smoking associated with sleep difficulty. Science 1980;207:551–53.

Strohl KP, Hensley MJ, Saunders NA, et al. Progesterone administration and progressive sleep apneas. JAMA 1981;245(12):1230–32.

Tilkian AG, Guilleminault WC, Schroeder JS, et al. Sleep-induced apnea syndrome: prevalence of cardiac arrhythmias and their reversal after tracheostomy. Am J Med 1977;63:348–58.

Tilkian AG, Motta J, Guilleminault WC. Cardiac arrhythmias in sleep apnea. In: Guilleminault WC, Dement WC, eds. Sleep apnea syndromes. New York: Alan R. Liss, 1978:197–210.

Van den Hoed T, Kraemer H, Guilleminault WC, et al. Disorders of excessive daytime somnolence: polygraphic and clinical data for 100 patients. Sleep 1981;4:23–37.

Vogel GW. A review of REM sleep deprivation. Arch Gen Psychiatry 1975;32:749–61.

Vogel GW, Thurmond A, Gibbons P, et al. REM sleep reduction effects on depression syndromes. Arch Gen Psychiatry 1975;32:765–77.

Webb WB, Agnew HW. Are we chronically sleep deprived? Bull Psychonomic Soc 1975;6:47–48.

Weitzman ED. Disorders of sleep and the sleep-wake cycle. In: Isselbacher KJ, et al, eds. Update one: Harrison's principles of internal medicine. 9th ed. New York: McGraw-Hill, 1981:245–63.

Williams RL, Karacan I, Hursch CJ. Electroencephalography (EEG) of human sleep: clinical applications. New York: John Wiley & Sons, 1974.

Zarcone V. Narcolepsy. N Engl J Med 1973;288:1156–66.

Zorick F, Roth T, Salis P, et al. Insomnia and excessive daytime sleepiness as presenting symptoms in nocturnal myoclonus. In: Chase MH, Mitler M, Walter PL, eds. Sleep research. Los Angeles: Brain Information Service/Brain Research Institute, UCLA, 1978;7:256 (abstract).

CHAPTER 6

Sleep Disorders in Infants and Children
Richard Ferber

For the past few years many sleep disorders clinics have been attempting to classify diagnoses according to nosological criteria developed by the Association of Sleep Disorders Centers (ASDC) (1979) (see Table 5.1 on page 82). This nosology was developed mainly from experience with adults and somewhat from experience with adolescents and older children, but only slightly from experience with infants and young children. As a result, there are some deficiencies regarding the younger groups. Nevertheless, an attempt is made here to follow the general ASDC nosology, extending it when necessary to include categories for younger children. The four general categories are: disorders of initiating and maintaining sleep (DIMS); disorders of excessive somnolence (DOES); disorders of the sleep-wake schedule; and dysfunctions associated with sleep, sleep stages, or partial arousals (parasomnias).

DISORDERS OF INITIATING AND MAINTAINING SLEEP (THE INSOMNIAS)

Early Infancy: Colic

The principal sleep disorder present during the first six months of life, except for the sudden infant death syndrome, is that associated with colic. Hence it is formally a disorder secondary to a medical condition, although its etiology is not fully understood. A colicky infant is irritable, with frequent, often inconsolable periods of crying especially in the afternoon and evening. The child appears to be in true distress and the origin is usually presumed to be gastrointestinal. Passage of flatus or feces may seem to relieve symptoms. Rocking, use of a pacifier, or application of warmth may bring some relief. Symptoms may be so marked that the pediatrician will try medication (phenobarbital, dicyclomine) with variable success. At bedtime and after nighttime waking, sleep onset is often delayed and accomplished only after extended periods of being held, rocked, or nursed. After the first three months, symptoms usually improve considerably and are rarely present beyond 6 months of age. At this point colic no longer seems a cause of sleep disturbance; however, patterns that developed during that period may continue so that the child may still sleep poorly (Illingworth, 1951). Thus, although no longer in pain, the child may be unable to fall asleep at bedtime or to return to sleep after nighttime wakings unless rocked or nursed. Furthermore, after helping a child through months of apparent suffering, it is difficult for a parent suddenly to ignore bedtime crying, to be convinced that the crying is now out of habit and no longer distress, and to set appropriately firm limits. These are actually some of the many factors that may affect the sleep of all infants or toddlers, not just those children who initially had sleep problems.

Older Infancy and the Toddler Years

In a frequently quoted paper, Moore and Ucko (1957) reported studying 160 British children longitudinally from birth for a period of one year. Settling was defined as regularly sleeping through the night from midnight until 5 AM for at least a four-week period. Seventy-one percent of babies did this by 3 months of age, 84 percent by 6 months, and 90 percent by 10 months. Ten percent never settled completely at any time during the first year. Various patterns were noted. Some infants gradually decreased the nighttime wakings, others settled suddenly as the 2 AM feeding was stopped, still others progressively woke at later times, and some were erratic in their pattern. The same authors also noted that 43 percent of those babies who initially settled subsequently reverted to nighttime wakings at some point, usually between ages 6 and 9 months. Thus whereas at 3 months only 20 percent were waking at night three or more times per week, and less than 2 percent were waking more than once nightly, in the second half-year these figures were approximately 32 percent and 13 percent respectively (Table 6.1, Figure 6.1). Ragins and Schachter (1971), who found that 55 percent of children settled by 2 months of age, also reported that nearly half of these showed increased waking in the second half-year. This increase in wakings between 6 and 12 months has also been noted by other investigators (Shepherd, 1948; Beal, 1969), but not all (Bernal, 1973). Carey (1974) found that 25 percent of children 6 to 12 months of age had periods of waking and crying one or more times a night between midnight and 5 AM at least four times per week for four or more consecutive weeks.

Even in the second year, problems persist. Bernal (1973) found that 27 percent of 14-month-old babies were still waking regularly at night. Richman (1981), in a survey of 1,000 children between ages 1 and 2 years, found 24 percent were still waking two to four times a week, and 9.5 percent were considered to have a severe disturbance that was defined as symptoms last-

Table 6.1. Distribution of Initial Settling and Later Relapses during the First Year of Life (104 Infants)

Month of Life	First Settled				Onset of Relapse	
	Percent without Relapse	Percent with Later Relapse	Total (%)	Cumulative (%)	%	Cumulative %
1	11.5	7.7	19.2	19.2	0	0
2	17.3	21.2	38.5	57.7	0	0
3	7.7	5.8	13.5	71.2	1.9	1.9
4	4.8	4.8	9.6	80.8	3.8	5.8
5	1.0	1.0	1.9	82.7	2.9	8.7
6	1.0	0	1.0	83.6	7.7	16.4
7	0	1.9	1.9	85.5	10.6	27.0
8	0	1.0	1.0	86.5	6.8	33.6
9	1.0	0	1.0	87.5	6.8	40.4
10	2.9	0	2.9	90.4	1.9	42.3
11	0	0	0	90.4	1.0	43.2
12	0	0	0	90.4	0	43.2
Totals	47.1	43.3	90.4		43.2	

Reprinted with modifications, by permission of the publisher, from Moore and Ucko (1957).

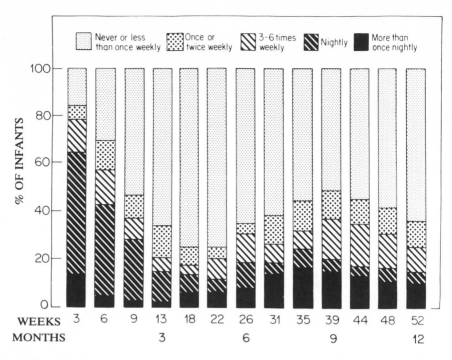

Figure 6.1. Incidence of night waking through the first year of life (104 infants). (Reprinted with modifications [data combined from two studies] by permission of the publisher, from Moore and Ucko, 1957.)

ing over three months with over five nights with wakings each week plus at least one of the following: three or more wakings a night, wakings lasting over 20 minutes, or the child getting into the parents' bed. Ragins and Schachter (1971) found 15 percent of 2-year-olds resisted bedtime, 10 percent suffered from problems of night wakings with difficulty returning to sleep, 44 percent had sleep problems of some concern to parents, and 12 percent were sleeping in the parents' room (all of these were children with regular wakings). Bax (1980) reported 20 percent of 2-year-olds were still waking to the point of disturbing the family. Finally, Roberts and Schoellkopf (1951), in a survey of over 750 2 1/2-year-olds, found 21 percent with one or more of five significant bedtime or sleep problems (most often resistance at bedtime) and 33 percent had at least some degree of disturbed sleep.

It is worth keeping in mind that by nighttime wakings, most authors are defining not just wakings per se but those that are abnormal because of their frequency, unusual features, subsequent delays in return to sleep, and demands for external intervention. Just as the sleep of most adults is interrupted by several brief awakenings on most nights, small children also wake normally. Anders (1979), for example, studying 2- and 9-month-old infants in the home with video recording found that only 44 percent of the children at 2 months and 78 percent at 9 months actually slept through without "apparent" waking (they were not monitored polygraphically so actual awakenings likely were even more frequent) between 10 and 5 AM. Only 6 percent at 2 months and 16 percent at 9 months went through the entire recording period without apparent awakenings. This is quite important because, as will be seen, what is often described by a parent as an "abnormal waking" is almost certainly normal, with the abnormality being in the delay in return to sleep. "Sleeping through . . . does not mean sleeping without awakening" (Anders, 1979). Anders also made the interesting and relevant observations that only about 60 percent at each age group were put into the crib awake, that parents still responded to nighttime wakings 33 percent of the time when the child was age 9 months, and only 55 percent of these 9-month-old infants were not removed at all from the crib during the night.

Since bedtime difficulties and nighttime disturbances between 6 months and 3 years of age are quite common, it might be tempting to accept them as normal developmental features. Several observations, however, suggest they best be considered a true disorder. First of all it has been noted (Moore and Ucko, 1957) that certain factors such as an illness could briefly interrupt a sleep pattern during the first three months of life without lasting effect, but later in the year a similar insult could lead to problems lasting for many months; in other words, in the second half-year a disrupting influence could have long-term effects. Environmental factors have also been shown to be important for settling. It has been observed that children born to mothers with at least two previous children settled significantly earlier than did first or second children (i.e., effect of maternal experience) and that there was increased waking and delayed settling among those who received less than 10 minutes or over 20 minutes per nursing (supposedly, where maternal-child interaction was poor or "oversolicitous"). Only 13 percent of babies who were not fed when they wakened at nighttime failed to settle by 13 weeks, as against 32 percent of those fed regularly and 40 percent who were fed variably. Weaning, in fact, seemed to lead to settling in some children, but never to increased waking; however, Bernal (1973) did not find such an association. In the 1- to 2-year-olds studied by Richman (1981), wakers still were more likely than nonwakers to use a bottle and probably also a pacifier at night, they were more likely to be the first child, and their mothers were more likely to have psychiatric disturbances.

Finally, there is evidence that physiologically different or damaged children settle later and wake more frequently (Moore and Ucko, 1957). This was true in children with increased daytime irritability and in those suffering asphyxia at birth. Of the latter group, 47.5 percent had not settled by age 3 months whereas only 28 percent of those with normal deliveries had not yet settled. Furthermore, the abnormal group continued with increased awakenings throughout the first year. The association of sleep disorders in the first year with birth asphyxia has been described by others

(Preston, 1945). Bernal (1973) noted that babies waking at age 14 months had a history of longer labor, took longer to cry after delivery, and had a lower score on a scale analogous to the Apgar than did controls. Richman (1981) found that 30 percent of 1- to 2-year-old children with sleep disturbances were considered at risk because of perinatal events versus only 16 percent of controls. Richman also pointed out that sleep difficulties in some of these toddlers could be due more to persisting altered dynamics between parents and children who survived a perinatal insult than to the direct effects of the insult itself.

In summary, despite the frequency of nighttime awakenings and bedtime difficulties in the population aged 6 or 9 months to 3 years, we consider this to represent a disorder because of the increase in symptoms in patients with some degree of neurological compromise, in families with less experienced parents, in situations with increased parental anxiety or psychiatric illness, in children with emotional problems (Fraiberg, 1950), and in families in which the parents are oversolicitous (Moore and Ucko, 1957; Richman, 1981). Learned habits associated with nighttime wakings (Illingworth, 1951, 1966; Richman, 1981), failure to "learn" to fall asleep without intervention after normal nighttime wakings (Bax, 1980), failure to establish proper diurnal rhythms (Kleitman, 1949), and inappropriate napping (Illingworth, 1951) are some of the other factors that have been considered significant.

Most important, perhaps, has been experience we have gained working with approximately 400 families with infants in this age range with a variety of bedtime difficulties and nighttime awakenings (Ferber, 1985; Ferber, Boyle, and Belfer, 1981a,b; Ferber and Boyle, 1983a–e; and unpublished data). Some of the factors described, plus other factors, could usually be identified and most often they were amenable to (usually behavioral) intervention with marked improvement of the sleep problem. This resolution was taken as further evidence that the patient's sleep disturbance was not a necessary developmental feature and was quite susceptible to satisfactory manipulation. As Richman has said, "Only by studying changes in children's sleeping patterns when the parents' management is changed or through a prospective study could one see how parents' behaviors are actually influencing sleep patterns" (1981).

Factors affecting the sleep of a young child are summarized in Table 6.2. Even when the underlying cause would best be classified as a disorder of the sleep-wake rhythm or at times as a parasomnia, the complaint is still usually one of bedtime difficulties or nighttime awakenings.

Inappropriate Associations with Sleep Transitions

Adults, children, toddlers, and infants all learn to associate the transitions to sleep with certain environmental factors such as a particular blanket, pillow, or side of the bed. Adults with insomnia may have negative associations with the bedroom but be able to fall asleep rapidly on the couch. Young children may have negative associations with the crib, but more as

Table 6.2. Factors Associated with Bedtime Difficulties and Nighttime Wakings in Infants and Toddlers

Etiological Factor	Closest ASDC Nosological Categories
	DIMS
Inappropriate associations with sleep transitions	Psychophysiological
Excessive fluid intake at night	Environmental conditions, psychophysiological
Poor and inconsistent limit setting	Environmental conditions*
Social factors	Psychophysiological, psychiatric disorders, subjective complaint without objective findings
Anxieties and fears	Psychophysiological, psychiatric disorders
Medical factors	Medical conditions
Central dysfunction	Medical conditions, childhood-onset
Medication	Use of drugs
	PARASOMNIAS
Sleepwalking, sleep terror, confusional arousals	Sleepwalking, sleep terror†
	SLEEP-WAKE SCHEDULE DISORDERS
Irregular sleep-wake pattern	Frequently changing sleep-wake schedule
Regular but inappropriate sleep-wake schedule	Not otherwise specified
Delayed sleep phase	Delayed sleep phase syndrome

*There is no category for the child who is trying to stay awake.
†Confusional arousals are not listed in the nosology.

a place where they do not want to be than as a place that is unpleasant because of time spent there unable to fall asleep. Still, they may have only learned to fall asleep elsewhere, especially in a parent's lap, being rocked, or nursing. They are placed in the crib asleep and when a normal awakening occurs later during the night they cannot simply return to sleep on their own. They will cry, but when a parent recreates the circumstances present at the initial sleep transition they calm rapidly and return to sleep.

Treatment, therefore, is straightforward. Children must learn to fall asleep under the same set of circumstances that will be present later at the time of spontaneous wakings (Douglas and Richman, 1982; Ferber and Boyle, 1983e; Ferber, 1985). Asking parents to simply let a child cry himself to sleep is not the best approach (Jones and Verduyn, 1983). It emphasizes the crying rather than the practice of falling asleep alone. Initially the child may cry for hours and eventually parents will give in, pick the child up, and allow him to fall asleep under the old conditions. If this happens, all the crying is wasted. A better approach, and one which leads to faster resolution of the sleep problem, lets the parents go to their crying child to briefly reassure him (and themselves) after progressively longer periods of waiting (Ferber, 1985). The waiting time may be only a few minutes initially but should increase between successive interventions and on successive nights. If absolutely necessary, a parent may sit by the bed at bedtime and after nighttime wakings. Then, over a period of several days, the chair may be gradually moved farther from the bed and out into the hall.

Excessive Fluid Intake at Night

Infants not given a bottle or immediately offered the breast when they wake at night may settle earlier than those who continue to be fed (Moore and Ucko, 1957; Elias et al, 1983), and 1- to 2-year-old wakers are more likely to use a bottle at night than are children who sleep through the night (Richman, 1981). Although the nighttime feeding could be in response to an existing sleep disorder, it is probably more often true that the feeding itself is the cause of the disorder (Ferber and Boyle, 1983c). Increased feeding at night may be a continuation from earlier infancy or represent a habit established after a transient sleep disturbance. In any case, a child who is nursing at the breast repeatedly during the night or who is receiving a full bottle at bedtime and then four to eight ounces more at each of four to seven nighttime wakings has a severe sleep disorder, but one that is easy to correct. Here the awakenings are not simply physiological but are increased most likely because of wetting, learned expectations of feedings, possible gastrointestinal and endocrinological effects of caloric and volumetric intake, and disruption of underlying circadian rhythms by the multiple arousals themselves. In a manner analogous to the adult who is sleeping poorly because of a sleeping medication taken in an effort to improve sleep, the child sleeps poorly because of the fluid given to aid each return to sleep. Although the child does get back to sleep each time, the total sleep pattern becomes quite disrupted. Gradual weaning of nighttime fluid, and if necessary that given to bed and nap times as well, leads to prompt resolution of this situation (Ferber and Boyle, 1983c; Ferber, 1985).

Poor and Inconsistent Limit Setting

What may perhaps seem to be the most obvious cause of sleep difficulties in young children is poor and inconsistent limit setting, but when actually faced clinically, the situation may be less clear-cut. The child, by a variety of verbal ("I want a glass of water") or behavioral (tantrums, looking cute, wanting to be held) tactics will make it clear that he or she would prefer to be somewhere else than bed. If the request seems minor, it may be hard to say no ("one more story, please") and if the consequences are pronounced (vomiting, even breath holding) it may also be difficult to be firm. If the complaint is a need to void or a fear of monsters, one may be unsure that the child's needs are not "real." As a result, the parent gives in. If this happens night after night it becomes an expected part of the bedtime routine and, in fact, the parents' failure to take control may be a true source of anxiety for the youngster who either is allowed to stay up and basically set his own place and time of retiring or to escalate his demands until some limit is finally set. But even when this limit is finally set, it is done inconsistently and in different manners on different nights with varying severity. The child may not know if on a given night he will end up in the parents' bed "cuddling" or in his own with a spanking. This too is a source of anxiety, which may be heightened if he is allowed into the parents' bed while one parent leaves to sleep elsewhere. Things are even more difficult (in terms of successful interventions) when the lack of limit setting actually has a parental motive, for example, when a mother prefers to have a child stay up with her at night ("for company") when her husband is working or when the child's presence "prevents" the parents from engaging in any form of intimacy.

Unlike most forms of "insomnia" in which the patient cannot sleep despite efforts to do so, in this situation (unless the secondary anxiety becomes sufficient) the child is perfectly capable of sleep but tries to avoid it, that is, he *will not* sleep rather than *cannot* sleep. If limits can be firmly and consistently set, resolution of the sleep problem will follow rapidly. To do this it will be necessary to determine if social issues are significant, and if so, these must be faced. Otherwise parents should institute a specific bedtime ritual at an appropriate time with a definite end point. One should negotiate with the parents a program that they can carry out of gradually increasing limit setting (e.g., amount of time of crying before intervention or amount of time with the door closed). There should be close follow-up and support necessary to help the family deal with the frequently faced feelings of guilt and anger. These interventions will usually bring resolution within one to two weeks. If the child is old enough, positive reinforcers such as a star chart for cooperation may also be therapeutic.

Social Factors

Social factors are complex, with the final common pathway to sleep disturbance usually through other factors discussed, such as lack of limit setting or patient anxiety. It is included here separately because despite the severity of the complaint, the actual degree of the disorder may be minimal, and because intervention has to be aimed at the social circumstances. Usually this means working with the parents, possibly involving them in counseling or therapy. Any source of stress at home may be responsible, including marital discord, alcoholism, affective illness, medical problems, financial difficulties, a family move, birth of a sibling, or a death. The presenting complaint, however, is of a sleep disorder, not of altered family dynamics. Careful work over a period of several weeks may be necessary to clarify the nature and degree of the sleep disturbance (e.g., sleep charting) and to form sufficient alliance with the family to begin facing the underlying issues directly. Depending on the specifics of the sleep disturbance, some direct efforts (such as normalizing the sleep schedule and improving bedtime rituals) may be useful while social efforts proceed.

Anxieties and Fears

Toddlers typically express their fears as being of the dark or of monsters. The underlying factors responsible for these fears usually have to do with issues of separation, concerns over loss of control, sibling rivalry, or specific psychosocial events such as overheard parental arguing, observed sexual acts, or the death of a relative or pet. Frequent actual nightmares or fear of such dreams conceivably may be a source of sleep disruption in this age group although it is difficult to document, especially in the preverbal child, and this is perhaps overestimated as a major cause of sleep disruption. Unless failure of limit setting is the main factor leading to increased anxiety, firmer limits run the risk of actually increasing the degree of panic. Intervention depends on a careful understanding of the underlying issues. If the child is otherwise functioning well and the concerns expressed are simply indicative of the normal psychological struggles characteristic of the present developmental stage, the problem should resolve spontaneously. Explanation and reassurance to the family will still be helpful and may avoid turning a transient disturbance into a chronic one. If the symptoms are already more pronounced or long-standing, further intervention is needed. If the factors are relatively minor they can be overcome by changing the pattern of parent-child interaction during the day and at bedtime routines. If the issues are more significant therapeutic aid for parents and/or child may become necessary (Fraiberg, 1950).

Medical Factors

Although medical factors should always be considered, they rarely are responsible for nighttime sleep disruption except in cases that are fairly obvious, for example, during an acute or subacute illness (upper respiratory tract infection, asthma) or with chronic discomfort such as in atopic dermatitis. In certain instances, however, the child may wake at night crying as if in pain and be difficult to calm regardless of parental response. If the child seems alert at these times and especially if some of these wakings occur toward morning, these events are unlikely to be sleep terrors. (Even if some of the events do suggest sleep terrors, a painful trigger must be considered.) If no illness or source of pain is obvious, the gastrointestinal and otolaryngological systems should still be considered and carefully evaluated. Either gastroesophageal reflux or chronic serous otitis media may lead to significant sleep disruption; frequent regurgitation or acute otitis does not have to be present. Treatment of these disorders may be followed by prompt resolution of the sleep problem. Usually medical therapy is sufficient, but occasionally surgery (fundoplication, tympanostomy tubes) is necessary.

Central Dysfunction

Settling of children with birth trauma is delayed and the incidence of waking in the toddler years remains increased. Thus one must consider whether the difficulties at age 2 are secondary to persistent central dysfunction or to other factors such as described elsewhere in this section that may have occurred because of the earlier difficulties. These factors are almost certainly responsible in certain instances, and helping a parent, for example, set firmer limits may resolve a problem completely despite history of neurological insult.

On the other hand, we have seen a number of children with mental retardation who have significant neurological deficits including severe sleep disorders for which scheduling or behavioral etiologies could not be identified. In these children there may be very little nocturnal or daytime sleep. Although sleep patterns may prove to be abnormal, with irregularly formed and poorly differentiated sleep stages, poor correlation of sleep parameters, and absent spindles, these findings do not explain why sleep is so short. Underlying seizure activity must be considered, although it is usually not the cause. If other factors are even suspected they should be treated first, and sometimes the results are surprisingly good. When they are not present or when behavioral modifications are ineffective, our assumption has been that these children have a true central dysfunction of sleep maintenance and/or of initiation, and it is in this group only that we have found medication to be useful. In most cases, chloral hydrate in substantial doses (e.g., 1–2 gm) has been useful without any evidence of daytime residua (daytime function may be improved) and often without evidence of tachyphylaxis despite prolonged therapy, although double-blind protocols have not yet been carried out. Small doses may not be beneficial at all and in fact may make things worse.

Medication

Chronic medication can be deleterious to the sleep of children as well as to that of adults. We have seen children, even infants, receiving medication for many months for what was thought to be a sleep disorder that resolved promptly on discontinuation of the agent. There are few situations in which an otherwise normal child would be expected to improve with regular use of any sleep medication, and in general such treatment should be carefully avoided. Even acute administration of a drug with sedating properties to a child may have paradoxical effects, that is, the child may remain awake and appear overactive, in the manner of a child overtired because of insufficient sleep.

Nonsedating medications also may disrupt sleep. Almost any drug has the potential to do this in a given child. Bronchodilators and other stimulants are especially notorious in this regard. If a child's sleep disturbance seems to have a pharmacologic basis, and if medication must be continued, then a change in drug, dosage schedule, or route of administration may still be helpful.

Sleep Terrors, Confusional Arousals, and Sleepwalking

Sleep terrors, confusional arousals, and sleepwalking are discussed mainly under the parasomnias but are mentioned here because in this age range the complaint is again simply nighttime waking. Bedtime is usually no problem but the child wakes crying one to three hours after falling asleep. Since intense crying, poor responsiveness, and failure or inability to report dream content verbally are expected at this age, the event is usually described as a bad dream or as another awakening.

True sleepwalking can also occur even in a toddler confined to the crib. It is interesting to note that Anders (1979), studying night waking in 9-month-old infants, found that both males and females showed the same peak time of awakening between 3 and 6 AM, but only males showed a second peak between 9 AM and midnight. Arousal symptoms such as night terrors are more common in males and one can only speculate that this finding is related to an instability in delta sleep. Roberts and Schoellkopf (1951) also reported that night terrors or bad dreams, crying out at night, or sleepwalking occur in about 30 percent of 2 1/2-year-olds and in 9 percent are significant enough to be considered a problem by the family.

Irregular Sleep-Wake Patterns

Although the underlying reasons may be varied, including lack of limit setting, social disruption, and cultural habits, some children are given poor structure for their daily routine. Bedtimes, nap times, times of morning awakening, and mealtimes vary from day to day. Disorganization of underlying circadian rhythms follows and sleep deteriorates. Nighttime sleep may be poorly consolidated. Daytime naps are irregular. They may occur late one day and interfere with sleep onset that night. On another day the naps may be missed and the child will retire early but awaken several hours later, having treated the early bedtime as a very late nap time. Total sleep time may be reduced. Initial attempts at an appropriate bedtime will fail because of the disturbance in sleep rhythms.

Although some children may tolerate varied patterns better than others, a regular daily routine is very important and should be listed at the top of any list of general rules for sleep hygiene in pediatrics. As Kleitman (1949) said, "The general requirement . . . is the maintenance of regularity in the daily schedule of feeding, bathing, play, etc., after the primitive 'self-demand' has been tempered by acculturation." Unless social factors interfere, most families, with guidance, can normalize their child's schedule (a sleep chart is extremely helpful). Even if sleep is difficult to enforce at first, time of waking is not (or at least it is easier). If the child awakens at a regular time, daily routines are consistent, and "sleep" time is spent as a quiet period, then the pattern will gradually normalize. If other disrupting factors are operative as well, they may need attention; but if sleep-wake rhythms are initially very disrupted, they should be corrected as the first goal.

Regular but Inappropriate Sleep-Wake Schedule

An inappropriate sleep-wake pattern may take several forms. A child who naps regularly at 4 PM may have difficulty falling asleep until 9 or 10 PM. Similarly, a child who continues to nap twice a day with the first nap occurring at 8 or 9 AM may be waking at 5 AM apparently wide awake and unwilling and unable to return to sleep. In this second case the last few hours of morning sleep have become separated from the nighttime sleep and appear several hours later as an unusually early morning nap. Eliminating this morning nap and moving the afternoon nap to right after lunch instead of the late afternoon may lead to consolidation of nighttime sleep with later morning awakening.

An inappropriately eliminated nap may also lead to sleep disturbance. Often the family of a child who is not sleeping well for whatever cause, even a transient one, may eliminate the nap in an attempt to improve sleep. Rather than improving, however, the child's sleep may deteriorate further with more difficulties at bedtime and/or further awakenings during the night. Since the child may not appear obviously sleepy during the day, the family does not realize that elimination of the nap actually made things worse. It is likely that this sleep-deprived youngster is operating under stress that negatively affects nighttime sleep. Reinstitution of regular napping times may lead to an increase in nighttime sleep rather than to a decrease. As is well known in folk wisdom, "one good sleep brings on another."

Delayed Sleep Phase

A child's sleep phase is that part of his circadian sleep-wake cycle in which sleep is most likely to occur. When the timing of this potential sleep period is later (delayed) than the patient and family want, the child will have difficulty falling asleep and waking until times later than desired (Weitzman et al, 1981).

When a delayed sleep phase occurs, there is a nightly bedtime struggle lasting several hours. Unlike the situation of poor limit setting described, however, the child does not sleep even if firm limits are set, if he gets into the parents' bed, or if a parent joins the child in his. Once asleep there usually are no nighttime wakings. Since sleep onset is delayed (and often because the parent likes to sleep late) the child is allowed to sleep late in the morning. Total sleep is adequate. If the child retires late, the sleep transition is rapid without a struggle. In this case it is true that the child is not falling asleep at bedtime because he *cannot,* not because he *will not*— he is not sleepy yet.

Physiological readiness for sleep, *Schlafbereitschaft* (Kleitman, 1949), has not yet arrived. His sleep cycle has been allowed to shift several hours later than desired, at least regarding bedtimes (Ferber, 1985; Ferber and Boyle, 1983d).

Treatment at this age is usually easy. Parents are told that the child cannot both go to sleep early and awaken late. If the early bedtime is chosen, an appropriately early time of morning waking eventually must be enforced seven days a week. An initially late bedtime can help remove the association of bedtime with struggles; this then, and the time of morning waking, can be gradually advanced, for example, 15 minutes every one to two days.

General Approaches to Management

In approaching the young child with sleep disruption it is important to take a detailed medical, developmental, and social history because of the many factors that may be relevant. Bedtime rituals should be understood, the exact pattern of parental intervention clarified, and the child's 24-hour sleep-wake and activity patterns carefully documented (Bax, 1980). Charting of sleep patterns over several weeks is extremely important either to obtain baseline information or to aid in carrying out and interpreting planned intervention. Objectivity of reporting nighttime events is quite difficult even when the family is well intentioned and cooperative; however, an irregular sleep pattern will be quite evident when charted, and the family will often find it easier to follow through on programs when the chart shows tangible evidence of success. General measures such as institution of a nonstimulating bedtime ritual in the child's room, avoiding the use of the bedroom as a place of punishment, and environmental manipulations such as use of a night light or leaving the bedroom door open may be helpful.

Although probably any child's sleep can be disrupted by certain environmental or physiological factors, it almost certainly is true that some children are much more resistant than others. Thus one child may fall asleep at bedtime being rocked and nursed, yet be able to fall back asleep alone in the crib after nighttime awakenings, whereas another child may only be able to return to sleep during the night if all such transitions, including bedtime, are made alone in the crib. Therefore few rules should be considered absolute. If things are working, the child is sleeping, and the family is happy, there is little motivation to urge change. When things are not going well, the family may be under great stress and intervention becomes urgent. It is important that the parents understand that a given pattern of interaction does not invariably lead to sleep disturbance, and hence their pattern of interaction was not necessarily "wrong," but a sleep disturbance depends on factors contributed by the child as well, and that only with full understanding can proper adjustments be assured. The interventions necessary to correct the sleep disorders are often difficult for parents to determine and carry out without advice, and little is gained by making them feel guilty or inadequate (Illingworth, 1951).

Prelatency and Latency

Complaints of difficulties falling or remaining asleep are much less common in the child aged 4 to 12 than in younger children. This is partly because the incidence of disturbances most likely is in fact reduced and also because the parents, who no longer are responsible for the child's every waking moment, may be unaware of sleep difficulties. A 9-year-old who is not falling asleep well may read in bed or lie and think without necessarily disturbing his parents; however, insomnia (usually sleep onset) may be present and be severe enough to cause the youngster distress. A sleep phase delay is possible but less likely at this age because school attendance forces early waking at least five days a week. Medical and neurological factors may be present and can be subtle. Irregular sleep-wake patterns are less common at this age than in the toddler and adolescent.

It is true, however, that most children at this age who are not falling asleep well at bedtime seem to be having worries or fears of varying degrees. Concerns such as about masturbation or about aggressive impulses toward family members may be present and, if not excessive, should be accepted as normal and handled with reassurance. Fears of dying while asleep may also arise, and the related anxiety is best relieved by frank discussions with care to distinguish sleep from death for the younger patient (Ferber and Rivinus, 1979). Those children with a somewhat obsessive-compulsive personality may simply lie and worry in the manner of a neurotic adult. Intervention in these cases is not very clear-cut and depends on the degree of disturbance, both of sleep and of personality. Although experience using adult techniques such as progressive relaxation for young insomniacs is very limited (Weil and Goldfried, 1973), we suspect that they would be useful. (Such techniques, however, have certainly been used on young patients with other disorders such as cancer.) We have also felt that some psychotherapeutic intervention should be carefully considered. This is more clear-cut when emotional disturbance is obvious, and such children do show more insomniac symptoms (Dixon, Monroe, and Jakim, 1981).

In some children, however, even those without major emotional disturbance, fears become overwhelming at night. Although well behaved during the day, they may scream hysterically and act wildly if sent to their bedrooms. They may well be willing to accept punishment if it keeps them from being alone. Here again we favor therapeutic interventions since the unresolved issues from which this behavior stems deserve attention (e.g., parents' divorce, a fire in the home, car accident, sibling jealousies). Some behavioral modifications may be helpful, for example, allowing a light, not having the child be two floors away from the closest adult, or getting a fire alarm for outside the bedroom.

There is also the suggestion at this age, as in younger age groups, that some children do not sleep well because of a central dysfunction of mechanisms responsible for initiating and maintaining sleep. Hauri and Olmstead (1980) have described such a group whose sleep difficulties began before the age of 10 and persisted into adulthood as childhood-onset insomnia. When these patients were studied as adults and compared with controls, they were found to have abnormally long periods of REM sleep totally devoid of eye movements, but otherwise no physiological differences were noted. Psychological evaluation was basically equivalent in the two groups; however, the patients with childhood-onset disorders had a suggestion of "soft neurological involvement" with histories including dyslexia, hyperkinesis, or minimal brain damage. It remains to try and identify such children before adulthood, to see if physiological differences are present at that age, and to see if early therapy affects outcome. One study that compared hyperkinetic and normal children between the ages of 8 and 12 years (Busby, Firestone, and Pivik, 1981) found that despite the frequent observation that hyperactive children sleep less, the only differences in sleep values were an increase in REM latency and some increase in movement time in the hyperkinetic group. Other studies (Haig, Schroeder, and Schroeder, 1974; Luisada, 1969; Feinberg, 1974; Khan and Rechtschaffen, 1978) also showed few changes in this group with or without stimulant medication.

Adolescence

During adolescence, problems increase in general, and difficulty falling asleep is just one of them. Surveys suggest that between 10 and 15 percent of adolescents have significant difficulties falling asleep, and another 38 percent report occasional disturbances (Anders, Carskadon, and Dement, 1980; Price, Coates, Thoresen, et al, 1978; Hertzman, 1948; Korlath, Baizerman, and Williams, 1976). The causes may be psychological, psychiatric, physiological, or medical. Psychological factors include anxiety induced by ambivalence over growing up, school demands, sexual pressures and fantasies, and family tensions (Marks and Monroe, 1976; Ferber and Rivinus, 1980). At this age the number of things that may serve as potential sources of worry seems almost endless. The resultant insomnia is essentially that described as psychophysiological in adults with somatized tension, anxieties, and negative conditioning to sleep (Association of Sleep Disorders Center, 1979). More significant psychiatric disorders may also emerge during adolescence, and sleep disruption is often the first symptom, for example, schizophrenia, anorexia, and mania (Easson, 1979). Although early morning awakening may be a symptom of adolescent depression (Anders, Carskadon, and Dement, 1980), depressed teenagers, more frequently than adults, show symptoms of hypersomnolence (Oswald, 1975). Medical factors such as beginning thyroid dysfunction or menstrual irregularities may certainly interfere with sleep. So may any of the drugs, including alcohol, that are now so frequently overused in this age group.

Although it has been shown that delta sleep decreases in total amount during puberty (Williams, Karacan, and Hursch, 1974; Carskadon, Harvey, Duke, et al, 1980; Feinberg, 1974; Williams, Karacan, and Davis, 1972; Karacan, Anch, Thornby, et al, 1975), one cannot take this as evidence of a decreased drive into sleep since it has also been shown that there is a progressive increase in apparent sleepiness throughout adolescence, at least as measured by the multiple sleep latency test (Carskadon et al, 1980). Perhaps the most important physiological influences are those that have to do with the general sleep-wake rhythms. Although in one study it was found that "contrary to popular belief, adolescents' sleep practices seem relatively stable" with patients following the same schedule on weekends and week nights and insomniacs doing this even more so in an attempt to minimize their sleep disturbance (Anders, Carskadon, and Dement, 1980), our own experience has been that irregular sleep-wake patterns in this group are in fact quite common. Most frequently seen is the adolescent who stays up very late into the early morning hours on weekend nights, sleeps late in the morning on weekend days, possibly naps during weekend afternoons, and has great difficulty waking for school on weekdays. The "insomnia" is most marked on weekday nights when an earlier bedtime is tried.

There seem to be two main factors. The irregularity of the sleep pattern has so disrupted the underlying circadian rhythms that well-consolidated, refreshing, good sleep becomes impossible. Even if this is not true, the underlying rhythms have been shifted or delayed by several hours so that, although the patient may actually sleep quite well, it is only from 3 AM until noon. Adolescents who seem truly motivated are able to follow through on a program of enforced morning awakening seven days a week, with careful charting demonstrating a gradual advance of sleep onset. At this age, however, it becomes difficult if not impossible for parents to enforce such a routine, and patient motivation is often minimal. Progressively delaying the sleep phase around the clock may also be successful (Czeisler, Richardson, Coleman, et al, 1979), but even here patient motivation becomes critical. The most severe cases of sleep phase delay that we have seen have been in adolescents with symptoms of school refusal in whom the profound sleepiness in the morning is used as an excuse for being unable to attend school (Ferber and Boyle, 1983b).

If the complaint of insomnia comes from the adolescent who is motivated for improvement, much work can be done. If rhythm disturbances seem to be the cause, careful explanation, planning, and sleep charting can lead to marked improvement. In certain youngsters who may be tense without specific sources of anxiety, who may seem to have constitutional difficulties with sleep transitions, that is, childhood-onset insomnia (Hauri and Olmstead, 1980), and possibly also in others with specific though relatively mild anxiety, various behavioral interventions such as have been described for the treatment of insomnia in adults may be quite beneficial (Anderson,

1979; Hauri, 1977, 1978, 1979). These include instructions in sleep hygiene and the use of relaxation techniques and biofeedback. At times psychotherapy seems clinically the best choice, but unfortunately, formal referral is often refused by the teenage patient. Sometimes one may continue to work *scientifically* with the patient about the sleep problem, gradually form an alliance, begin to let the conversation wander to personal issues, and eventually begin, or refer for, formal therapy.

DISORDERS OF EXCESSIVE SOMNOLENCE

The main disorders of excessive sleepiness seen during childhood and adolescence are those of obstructive sleep apnea and narcolepsy. Other causes do exist, but those causing severe sleepiness are rare and in these cases a central dysfunction must be ruled out by complete neurological evaluation. Milder degrees of sleepiness or lethargy may be present with medical illness such as hepatitis, mononucleosis, anemia, leukemia, or other debilitating conditions. Menstrual-associated sleepiness (Billiard, Guilleminault, and Dement, 1975) or periodic hypersomnia associated with Kleine-Levin syndrome (Levin, 1936) are rare. Hypersomnia as a symptom of adolescent depression, however, is not infrequent and must be carefully ruled out (Oswald, 1975). Drug and alcohol abuse must be similarly considered.

Obstructive Sleep Apnea

The obstructive sleep apnea syndrome, in which there are repeated sleep-associated obstructions of the midpharyngeal airway leading to hypoxia, sleep disruption, and cardiovascular changes, is now well described in the adult literature (Guilleminault, 1976; Guilleminault, Korobkin, and Winkle, 1981; Guilleminault and Dement, 1978; Phillipson, 1979; Lugaresi, Coccagna, and Mantovani, 1978). It almost certainly represents the most frequent cause of pathologically excessive daytime sleepiness in adult males over the age of 40 years. It has been less well recognized, however, that basically the same syndrome exists throughout childhood. It is true that associations between adenotonsillar enlargement and cor pulmonale in children have been made on a number of occasions (Noonan, 1965; Menashe, Fearron, and Miller, 1965; Luke, Mehrizi, Folger, et al, 1966; Levy, Tabakin, Harrison et al, 1967; Massumi, Sarin, Pooya, et al, 1969; Talbot and Robertson, 1973; Bland, Edwards, and Brinsfield, 1969; Goodman, Goodman, Gootman, et al, 1976). More recently clear-cut demonstrations of complete sleep apnea syndromes with full polygraphic monitoring have been made (Guilleminault, 1976; Guilleminault, Korobkin, and Winkle, 1981; Mangot, Orr, and Smith, 1977; Kravath, Pollak, and Borowiecki, 1977, 1980; Guilleminault, Eldridge, Simmons, et al, 1976; Ferber, Friedman, and

Dietz, 1983e). As awareness is enhanced and diagnostic facilities become more available, the frequency with which this diagnosis will be made in children will continue to increase considerably. For example, Guilleminault et al (1981) recently reported on 50 children with obstructive apnea, and we (Ferber, Friedman, and Dietz, 1983e) recently described another 80 children with this disorder. Both groups have now treated more than 100 such patients.

The syndrome may be present at all age ranges, from infancy to adolescence, with specifics being somewhat age-dependent. Principal symptoms seen in the adult and in the child are summarized in Table 6.3. Very loud nocturnal snoring is universal, often has been present since early infancy, and may have increased gradually over the months and years, or acutely, following an episode of adenotonsillitis. Increase in symptoms accompanying an upper respiratory infection is common. Adolescents often show the marked daytime sleepiness typical of this syndrome in the adult; in younger children this may be quite subtle, appearing instead as hyperactivity, attentional difficulties, various behavior problems, and decreased school performance. The child's sleep may be restless, but sometimes despite obstructions it is surprisingly calm with thrashing absent. There seems to be a 3 : 2 male predominance (Ferber, Friedman, and Dietz, 1983e), much less marked

Table 6.3.   Features of Obstructive Sleep Apnea in Children and Adults

Findings and Symptoms	Adults	Children
Very loud nocturnal snoring	Always	Always
Daytime sleepiness	Often severe	Often subtle (hyperactivity, attentional deficits, other behavior problems, decreased school performance)
Nocturnal thrashing	Usual	Occasional
Sex predominance	95% male	Some increase in males (perhaps 60%)
Body habitus	Stocky to obese	Variable (normal, obese, failure to thrive)
Enuresis	Occasional	Common (primary or secondary)
Nightmares, sleep terrors	Uncommon	Occasional to frequent
Daytime systemic hypertension	Common	Uncommon
Morning headaches	Common	Occasional
Predisposing physical condition	Usually none (except obesity)	Usually present (most often tonsils and/or adenoids)
Automatic behavior	Common	Rare

than the male predominance noted for obstructive apnea in the adult (at least when men are compared to age-matched premenopausal women).

Most childhood patients, unlike adults, do demonstrate soft tissue or skeletal abnormalities of etiological importance. The most frequent association is with enlarged tonsils and/or adenoids. It is interesting that the syndrome may be present with only adenoidal enlargement, that is, when the oral airway is completely patent. Apparently these children have difficulty switching to mouth breathing during sleep. It is important to realize that the degree of adenotonsillar enlargement necessary to produce obstruction does not have to be overwhelming; even when tonsils are huge one cannot predict from physical examination alone what will be the respiratory effects during sleep. Furthermore, unless indirect mirror examination can be satisfactorily carried out, which is often difficult in a young child, the true extent of lymphoid hyperplasia may not be fully appreciated. Radiological examination may aid in such estimation. Other soft tissue compromise may also be responsible, such as that seen with tumor or fat infiltration (Hodgkin's disease, obesity) or with relative macroglossia (trisomy 20-Down's syndrome). Isolated retrognathia has frequently been associated with this disorder, as have other maxillofacial malformations (Crouzon's disease, Pierre Robin syndrome). The development of obstructive apnea following surgical creation of a pharyngeal flap for velopharyngeal incompetence has been seen, and at least one case ultimately resulted in fatality (Kravath et al, 1980). Associations with various neurological and neuromuscular disorders such as myotonic dystrophy, Chiari malformations, and the Shy-Drager syndrome have also been noted. Obesity is a common finding in adolescent patients as it is in adults, but especially in the younger patient normal habitus or actual failure to thrive may be present. Nocturnal enuresis, primary or secondary, is common among these children and there may be disruption of nighttime sleep with sleepwalking, sleep terrors, or nightmares. Daytime hypertension is not common in younger children, although it may be present in the adolescent, and electrocardiographical evidence of right ventricular hypertrophy may be found. Automatic behavior or sleep drunkenness is rarely reported. Although delta sleep may be markedly diminished, in many young children it persists and may even be completely adequate in total amounts; perhaps this is why these children show less daytime somnolence. When delta sleep is reached, obstruction usually decreases, being more profound, as expected, in stage II and especially in REM sleep. Morning headaches are not common, especially in the young. Some of these children, instead of showing complete obstructions, will continue to breath through a partial obstruction for extended periods, with retractions and obviously increased respiratory effort. During these times, levels of blood gases may remain normal or there may be some desaturation with arterial oxygen tension that either is maintained at a lower than normal but relatively constant level or gradually decreases over several minutes until stimulating an arousal. When such patterns are present in non-rapid eye movement (NREM) sleep they often convert to complete obstruction during rapid eye movement (REM) sleep.

There are some significant differences between the 50 cases reported by Guilleminault et al (1981) and those that we have seen in our center (Ferber, Friedman, Dietz, 1983e). Those described by Guilleminault showed more severe day and nighttime symptoms and more frequently had significant pathology not related to tonsils or adenoids. Furthermore, 20 percent of their patients had investigations for sleep apnea after emergency hospitalization for acute cardiac or cardiorespiratory failure. None of the children we have examined to date has demonstrated such distress. The majority were referred for evaluation from the otolaryngological department or (less often) from the weight-reduction clinic because of a history suggestive of obstructive apnea. In addition, three-quarters of our patients had significant adenotonsillar enlargement. A tracheostomy was required in only three cases; two of these were precautionary and both have already been closed. Of those reported by Guilleminault and associates, half had pathology not related to tonsils or adenoids, only one-fourth were considered to have mildly enlarged tonsils or adenoids, and only 4 patients had quite significant lymphoid enlargement. Nevertheless, 27 of their patients showed significant improvement or complete resolution of obstruction following removal of tonsils and adenoids, only 3 of 30 children so operated upon subsequently required a tracheostomy, and 5 other patients not so operated on required such surgery. Of our 80 patients, aged 14 months to 17 years (51 boys, 29 girls), 23 had both enlarged lymphoid tissue and other predisposing factors. Of these 23, 9 were markedly obese (3 had Prader-Willi syndrome) and 14 others showed various neurological or autonomic abnormalities. In all of these patients, removal of lymphoid tissue was helpful; in many of them there was total or near total resolution of obstruction. In the very obese, however, weight reduction was also necessary before respiration became normal.

Obstructive sleep apnea in adults is discussed in Chapter 5.

It is important to be aware that obstructive sleep apnea in children exists, is much more common than is generally realized, and is present at all pediatric ages. It is likely that the number of cases has increased in recent years because of trends away from removing pharyngeal lymphoid tissue. There has been a tendency on the part of physicians to ignore complaints of nighttime snoring in children when the awake child they are currently examining appears well, possibly completely normal, and without signs of respiratory embarrassment. Since snoring implies a partial obstruction of airflow, even if not yet associated with complete obstruction or hypoxia, it may be associated with increased respiratory effort, cardiovascular changes, sleep disruption, and altered daytime performance. A high index of suspicion, careful history (e.g., of the presence and character of snoring, sleepiness, behavioral changes, and enuresis), and general physical examination with careful evaluation of the upper airway and cardiovascular system are mandatory. Airway films or specialized maxillofacial radiographs, otolaryngological, craniofacial, and oral surgical consultative evaluations, and fiberoptic studies may be considered. Baseline electrocardiogram and possibly a chest x-ray may be important. Finally, if there is reasonable suspicion, a polysomnographic evaluation is important not simply to establish the diagnosis but to assess severity, which is important when planning and subsequently evaluating intervention.

Medical therapy is the least likely to be successful but may be considered in an effort to avoid surgery. Certainly, dietary treatment of obesity is a reasonable start. Of the obese patients we have seen, it is noteworthy that the most severe apnea has been in those who also had adenotonsillar enlargement. In these children, removal of the lymphoid tissue led to substantial if not complete resolution of symptoms even before subsequent weight loss. Pharmacological treatment with medroxyprogesterone, steroids, protriptyline, or acetazolamide may be useful in certain children (Guilleminault, Korobkin, and Winkle, 1981). Surgical procedures include, of course, removal of tonsils and adenoids, and if other approaches are not available, a tracheostomy. Orofacial surgery such as division of a previously constructed pharyngeal flap or advancement of a retrognathic mandible may be helpful. To date there is little experience treating children with uvulopalatopharyngoplasty surgery (UPPP) (Fujita et al, 1980, 1981, 1983; Silvestri et al, 1982) or nocturnal nasal continuous positive airway pressure (CPAP) (Rapoport et al, 1982; Sullivan et al, 1981), although the latter may prove useful as a temporary measure for the obese child during weight reduction. Finally, documented apnea in extremely obese patients who have failed to respond to dietary therapy may be used as evidence to support more urgent intervention such as gastric stapling and bypass surgery.

Narcolepsy

Narcolepsy occurs sporadically, with an incidence of about 0.4 percent, but is seen with much higher incidence, about 5 percent, within narcoleptic families (Kessler, 1976). A multifactorial mode of transmission is felt to be responsible, with variable penetrance.

Although some features of excessive sleepiness such as overactivity or continued napping may be seen in children who ultimately develop a full narcoleptic syndrome, major sleepiness or the development of other symptoms before adolescence is uncommon. The peak age of onset is between 15 and 25 years, with the most common early symptom being excessive sleepiness. Cataplexy, hypnagogic hallucinations, and sleep paralysis begin to appear after different intervals. In a restrospective study (Navelet, Anders, and Guilleminault, 1976), it was shown that in patients who had developed clear-cut narcolepsy, almost 50 percent had at least one symptom before age 16 and almost 20 percent had two symptoms before age 17. Five percent developed the complete syndrome before the end of the fifteenth year. Symptoms of sleepiness had been present at much earlier ages than previously recognized. Thus 20 percent of patients were considered "long sleepers" even in childhood, and almost half of the subjects continued to nap routinely after the age of 5. Significant complaints of daytime sleepiness began to appear between 5 and 15 years of age (mean, 11.5 years) and inappropriate napping slightly later (mean, 13 years). Hypnagogic hallucinations or repetitive nightmares were reported in 23 percent before age 17, with repetitive sleep paralysis being seen with the same frequency. Cataplexy was reported in only 16 percent by this age.

Now that there is increasing awareness of narcolepsy as a syndrome in adults, the diagnosis is being made earlier and with increased frequency, however, it is rarely before adulthood. Since these retrospective studies show some symptoms present even before adolescence, a high degree of suspicion becomes necessary. One problem is that when the only symptom is sleepiness, an early definitive diagnosis of this syndrome is not always possible. Before the development of cataplexy, a clinical diagnosis may be difficult and the laboratory finding of a sleep-onset REM period (SOREMP) may not yet be present. Still, full polysomnographic monitoring followed by multiple sleep latency testing is recommended. Even if SOREMPs are not present, the finding of short sleep latencies, which otherwise are quite unusual in latency and early adolescence, should be considered very significant.

A decision to use medication can be made on clinical grounds based on current symptoms, even if full laboratory documentation, except for short sleep latencies, is not present. If there is a family history of narcolepsy in a child with suggestive symptoms, or if the pattern of sleepiness is sufficiently characteristic (i.e., relatively short refreshing naps despite adequate nocturnal sleep) and the sleep latencies are short, then the diagnosis may be considered likely. Since narcolepsy is a lifelong disease, one should be cautious to make such a diagnosis definitely, and it is better to follow the child closely over the years waiting for more complete evolution of symptoms. Medication is basically the same as that used in adults, with stimulant therapy for the sleepiness and tricyclic medication for the associated symptoms.

RHYTHM DISTURBANCES AND INSUFFICIENT SLEEP

As suggested, both irregular sleep patterns and a sleep phase delay may lead to sleep cycle alterations, perhaps, although not necessarily, with decreased sleep and marked difficulty arising in the morning (Figure 6.2). At times this may be the main complaint. Similar etiological and treatment factors as described for insomnia apply here.

Insufficient sleep may be responsible at all ages, although this may not be obvious at initial interview. It is important to keep in mind that the overtired child may not appear sleepy but instead may show signs of over-activity, inattentiveness, impulsivity, and varying behavioral changes. Although such symptoms may customarily be associated with being overtired in a usually normally functioning child, when they are present constantly they may be ascribed to other etiologies. Most striking in this regard, perhaps, is the fact that many patients who were given the diagnosis of narcolepsy as adults had been treated with stimulants in childhood for "hyperactivity" (Navelet, Anders, and Guilleminault, 1976).

Carskadon et al (1980) suggested that increased sleepiness is an inherent part of the pubertal transition, intensified in our current society by insufficient sleep of a social etiology. They found that when adolescents were allowed to sleep at night in a controlled setting, total sleep time was about nine hours and there was a 40 percent reduction in delta sleep from prepuberty to maturity. Multiple sleep latency testing as a measure of sleepiness also suggested the development of significantly more sleepiness with increasing maturation, with peaks in the early and midafternoon. Increased sleepiness with decreased delta sleep, present even when the adolescent slept one and one-half hours more than usual, was seen as evidence that the observed increase in daytime sleepiness occurs both as a direct function of maturation and in response to some degree of sleep deprivation. The findings of Webb and Agnew (1975) are interesting in this regard, since they suggest that total sleep time in the adolescent has decreased about 90 minutes over the past 70 years.

PARASOMNIAS

Disorders of Arousal

Although sleep terrors, sleepwalking, sleeptalking, confusional arousals, and enuresis are often discussed as being separate entities, for this discussion it seems more appropriate to group all of them, except perhaps enuresis, together. This is because they all seem to be events that may accompany the termination of an episode of slow wave sleep.

In the normal sleep progression in children and adults, sleep onset is rapidly followed by descent into the deeper stages of NREM sleep, namely stage IV, where high-amplitude delta activity occupies almost the entire record. After an hour or so in this state there is usually a "slow wave arousal episode" (Broughton, 1968) during which there are a burst of semiregular high-amplitude delta activity, nonspecific body movements, and signs of

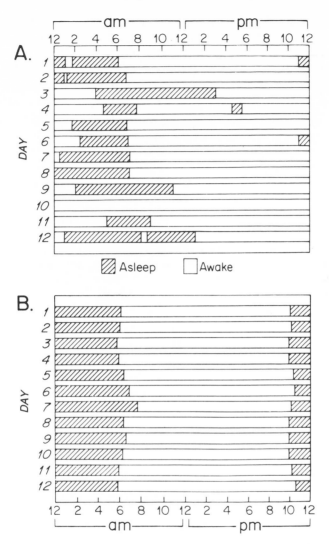

Figure 6.2. Sleep profile in a 16-year-old boy with a complaint of severe difficulty waking for school despite an honest desire to do so. Morning confusion (sleep drunkenness) was common. (A) Initially there was a very erratic sleep pattern with sleep onset between 11 PM and 5 AM, waking between 7 AM and 3 PM, total daily sleep usually between 4 and 11 hours, and one day with no sleep at all. (B) Very stable pattern with sleep onset at 10 PM and waking at 6 to 7 AM following institution of a program of regularized bedtimes and wakings seven days a week. The patient cooperated fully, morning awakenings were no longer a problem, and morning confusion disappeared.

arousal. This may be followed by transition into lighter stages of NREM, rapid return to stage IV, or even occasionally by an almost sudden transition into REM. In young children a REM episode at this point is usually missed, and after a brief time in stage II sleep another descent into stage IV occurs. In the adolescent this is also possible, but a brief REM period may intervene.

At the moment of the arousal from slow wave sleep, manifestations may sometimes be more marked. Body movements may be more exaggerated and extended in time and there may be some moaning or even nonspecific verbalization. The child may open his eyes briefly, look about with a glassy-eyed appearance, and seem to be unaware of anyone else's presence in the room. He may sit up, move about in a semiconfused manner, and fuss with sheets. Verbalization may be more prominent and usually only semicoherent. If the arousal is more pronounced the child may begin to whimper, cry, or thrash about (Figure 6.3), and/or get out of bed and begin to walk around. When there is walking, it may or may not be accom-

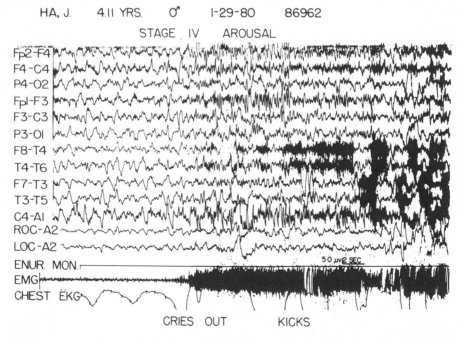

Figure 6.3. Confusional arousal in a boy 4 years 11 months old. There is progressive arousal with kicking, thrashing, and crying out but no screaming. The EEG shows fairly sudden arousal. There is even rapid reappearance of alpha rhythms, but they are not well localized to the posterior regions as they would be if the patient had reached full waking. Muscle artifact only partly obscures the record. This event lasted for about five minutes.

panied by those aspects more suggestive of a sleep terror. Walking may be aimless, possibly just around the room, or it may be down the hall and even downstairs. A frequent history that suggests both a confusional state and the need to urinate is wandering to a closet or to a corner and then urinating. With more pronounced arousals, the child may appear frightened and even terrified, screaming and sweating with heart racing. At these times he will be impossible to calm, will tend to push away anyone attempting to provide comfort, and will not even seem to recognize parents. In young children such states are usually reached gradually and may be quite prolonged, lasting anywhere from less than 1 minute to 30 minutes or more (Ferber and Boyle, 1983a). In the more prolonged events, when the child cannot be aroused, parents may be afraid and rush him to the hospital only to have the child wake on the way and be perfectly normal at the time of examination. In adolescents the sleep terror is more typical of that seen in the adult, beginning very suddenly with a scream, usually followed by broken phrases that suggest concern of attack ("It's going to get me," "I'm going to be crushed"), abandonment, aggression, or death (Fisher, Kahn, Edwards, et al, 1974), and ending after only seconds to several minutes (Figure 6.4). In the most marked episodes, seen more frequently in adolescents than in younger children, the patients not only will scream but will jump out of bed and run about wildly, usually as if to escape something. This is perhaps the reaction that puts the patient at greatest risk for self-injury, for he may jump out a window, fall down the stairs, or run out of the house and down the street.

During all these events, the high-amplitude, rhythmical delta activity that seems to represent the NREM arousal pattern (even similar patterns can be seen on sudden arousal from stage II where ongoing background is not in the delta range) gradually diminishes and the slow activity becomes mixed with faster rhythms suggestive of stage I or waking; at times, some return of alpha rhythms may even be seen (Fisher, Kahn, Edwards et al, 1973a,b) but with diffuse rather than posterior distribution. Clinically and electroencephalographically the patient seems to be in a dissociated state with simultaneous features of waking and NREM sleep. Even the visual evoked potential is intermediate between that expected for waking and slow wave sleep (Broughton, 1968).

There is little one can do to alter the course of these events. Attempts to hold, restrain, or comfort the child may intensify the episodes, but occasionally a child will seem to allow himself to be calmed. A calm sleepwalker probably will allow himself to be led to the bathroom and/or back to bed. Forced awakenings are almost impossible, especially during the most pronounced episodes. As the events terminate, the child will usually calm rapidly, relax, stretch, and yawn. He may be briefly alert, but will return to sleep almost instantly unless more fully wakened at this time by an anxious parent. If awakened, the young child almost always demonstrates total

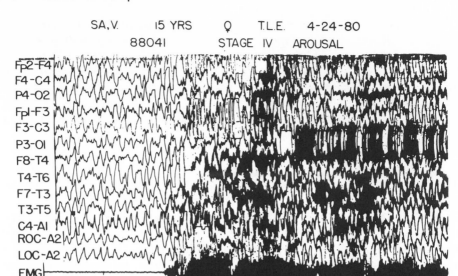

Figure 6.4. A sleep terror in a 15-year-old girl. There is an extremely sudden arousal with a scream and then a period of brief confusion lasting less than one minute, brief alerting, and return to sleep. The EEG shows delta rhythms on the left and then higher-voltage, more rhythmical delta during the arousal; much of the EEG during the arousal is obscured by muscle artifact.

amnesia for the event, whereas the adolescent may remember fleeting vague content in accord with the utterances just issued (i.e., he may still claim "something" was after him but be unable to elaborate).

That these events are not dreams is clear from the characteristics of the arousal: out of slow wave sleep with little or no imagery. Nightmares arise out of REM and are associated with imagery prolonged over time in a story fashion, that is, a succession of occurrences. The brief and vague nature of sleep terror utterances (and subsequent recall, if present), and the fact that similar arousals can be precipitated suddenly by touching susceptible patients, standing them up, or ringing a buzzer while they are in stage IV sleep (Broughton, 1968; Fisher et al, 1973; Kales, Jacobson, Paulson, et al, 1966) suggests that content is generated during rather than precipitating arousal. It may be, however, that the intensity of the arousal is related to the psychological state of the child. Thus a person afraid of attack, concerned with loss of control, or otherwise under stress might react differently to being in a dissociated state than might another person.

These arousal symptoms definitely have a genetic component, although the pattern of inheritance (or even what is inherited—for example, a tendency to sleep deeply or to arouse partially) is not clear. About 15 percent of children are said to have walked in their sleep on at least one occasion and only 1 to 3 percent to have had a sleep terror (Kales, Jacobson, and Kales, 1969). Our own experience and data from Roberts and Schoellkopf (1951), however, suggest that the incidence of sleep terrors is at least 15 percent as well. This depends somewhat on the strictness of the definition of sleep terror as compared with the milder confusional arousal and the care with which these arousals are differentiated from bad dreams. Abnormal NREM arousals are probably most frequently underdiagnosed in infants and toddlers as discussed above. Episodes of regularly occurring sleepwalking or sleep terrors, however, are certainly less common. Events are most common in the early years, are often most recognized in the 4- to 6-year-old group, and tend to decrease gradually thereafter.

Although it is clear that there may be an inherited tendency to such symptoms, and at times a known external stimulus can be identified, the usual arousal stimulus is not known. Only occasionally may pain (gastroesophageal reflux, arthralgia) be identified. Symptoms seem to be more frequent during an illness conceivably secondary to discomfort, to sleep rhythm disruption, or to increased drive to delta sleep. Increased symptoms specifically with a febrile illness have been described (Kales, Kales, Soldatos, et al, 1979) and we have had similar reports in our own patient population. Sleep disruption (fragmentation plus initially decreased delta sleep) has been associated with fever (Karacan, Wolff, Williams, et al, 1968) possibly followed by rebound increases in stages III and IV. Parents of our patients most frequently reported increased arousals when their children were "overtired," again suggesting more drive into delta sleep. Similarly, we have seen increased symptoms when naps were stopped or sleep was otherwise insufficient. Symptoms often abated when the amount of sleep was normalized.

It may be that the arousals do involve REM mechanisms (Arkin, 1978). It has been shown that REM rhythms are somewhat independent of those of NREM, the former being more closely linked to the underlying circadian rhythms and the latter to the onset of the sleep period itself; thus the REM latency may be shorter after a progressively later bedtime on a free-running schedule (Weitzman, Czeisler, Zimmerman, et al, 1980). In children, after termination of the first episode of stage IV there may be a brief period during which the electroencephalogram (EEG) begins to suggest REM, electromyogram (EMG) declines, but spindles and NREM return quickly, and another descent into slow wave sleep follows. It looks as if an unsuccessful attempt to establish fully formed REM had been made. This conceivably could represent the emergence of the basic rest-activity cycle with REM arousal mechanisms incompletely interrupting ongoing NREM and then giving way to the continued strong NREM pressure that is present early in the night. This remains to be tested; however, we have also seen arousal symptoms in children with quite irregular sleep-wake schedules and found the symptoms to disappear completely with no intervention other than regularization of the sleep pattern.

Psychological factors are clearly important to these episodes of sleep disruption. Several studies in adults claim that sleepwalkers are outwardly directed and have difficulties handling their aggression (Kales, Soldatos, Caldwell, et al, 1980; Sours, Frumkin, and Indermill, 1963), whereas those with sleep terrors are said to inhibit their aggression and tend to show elements of depression and obsessive-compulsive and phobic behavior (Kales, Kales, Soldatos et al, 1980). Both groups showed higher degrees of psychopathology than did controls. Among the adolescents whom we have seen in both groups, denial and repression of anger coupled with outward friendliness, placidity, and cooperative behavior or with silence, withdrawal, and passive-aggressive behavior have been the most common patterns.

One is generally correct in assuming that symptoms in early childhood are related to genetic, developmental, and scheduling problems, and symptoms that persist, recur, or first occur in latency or adolescence involve emotional factors even if there is genetic predisposition. Yet one must be aware that stress can lead to new or increased symptoms in toddlers as well. Similarly, the assumption that emotional factors are relevant in an adolescent with frequent recurrent symptoms should be verified clinically before intervention is planned.

In young children, sources of stress and physical discomfort must be considered before proceeding and be dealt with as indicated. If there is any suggestion of insufficient sleep, for example late bedtimes, or the inappropriate stopping of naps, these should be corrected. Finally, the child should be tried on a regular pattern of retiring and waking. The parents should be given a careful explanation of the events, told to "keep their distance" and be prepared to help only to the extent it is accepted, and let the child return to sleep as the events terminate without forced waking and questioning that may lead to more prolonged full waking and the generation of anxiety related to sleep. Morning questioning should be similarly avoided. The child has no memory for these episodes, and generating worry about the "strange things" he may do at night can only serve to increase symptoms. Although pharmacological treatment has been described, especially with diazepam (Fisher et al, 1973b) and imipramine (Pesikoff and Davis, 1971; Logan, 1979; Beitman and Carlin, 1979) they are rarely necessary and should be reserved for those whose symptoms are frequent, significantly disruptive to a poorly coping family, putting the child at risk for physical injury, and unresponsive to simpler behavioral manipulations. If medication is really necessary, we agree with Kales, Kales, Soldatos, et al (1980) and prefer to avoid diazepam in young children. The response to imipramine may be striking, although not necessarily so, and some children respond with poorer sleep and increased REM nightmares. In the adolescent, when emotional factors are clearly relevant and symptoms significant, psychotherapy is indicated. Drug suppression of episodes is important if the patient is at risk for injury but should not be used instead of psychotherapy; once progress has been made in therapy, tapering of medication can be begun. Either diazepam or imipramine may be tried, but if suppression is urgent, diazepam is recommended. To date there is little experience treating the arousal disorders with shorter-acting benzodiazepines. For patients of all ages, general management should include environmental changes so that the windows are locked and floors kept clear, and the patient should not sleep in an upper bunk. If he tends to leave the home, extra locks can be used, as can bells or buzzers that ring when the door opens to warn family members.

Enuresis

Enuresis is discussed separately because its relationship to stage IV arousals is somewhat unclear. Studies have shown that enuresis usually does in fact occur as part of an arousal from slow wave sleep in a manner similar to, although not as sudden as, that seen in sleep terrors and sleepwalking (Broughton, 1968; Pierce, 1963; Pierce, Whitman, Maas, et al, 1961; Saint-Laurent, Batini, Broughton, et al, 1963). Most episodes of enuresis do occur during the first third of the night when slow wave sleep is most plentiful. Furthermore, wetting may acompany a confusional arousal or sleep terror, and a sleepwalker may void inappropriately. In some children these arousals differ from night to night. Kales et al (1977), however, argue that enuresis is more related to the time of night than it is to particular sleep stage, that it is more common early in the night, with two-thirds of the episodes occurring in the first one-third of the sleep period, and for that reason it is most often associated with slow wave sleep. They say that enuretic events occur out of each sleep stage in approximate proportion to the time spent in that stage for each one-third of the night.

Thus sleep-related enuresis is complex, and different factors or mechanisms may be involved depending on the stage in which it occurs. Most enuresis does seem to occur as part of an arousal from slow wave sleep. True REM-associated enuresis is uncommon and hence dreams of wetting usually occur in REM periods after wetting has already taken place. Enuresis in the early morning, for example, may be less physiological and more behavioral, may occur in waking or light sleep, and may involve motivational factors (i.e., it being too cold to get out of bed).

It is clear, however, that there is a definite inherited tendency (Bakwin, 1973), with a positive family history frequently found, and that there is a higher incidence in males. Multiple studies have shown decreased functional bladder capacities in many enuretic children (Starfield, 1967; Vullaimy, 1956) but this finding is neither a necessary nor sufficient condition for enuresis.

Increased bladder contractions occurring spontaneously or in response to noise have also been described (Broughton, 1968; Broughton and Gastaut, 1964). Although it has been said that enuretics are deep sleepers, studies have not consistently been able to document this (McLain, 1979). If behavioral problems are more commonly found in the enuretic patient, they are only slightly so (Hallgren, 1958; Werry, 1967). Thus even persistence of enuresis into adolescence, unlike that of sleep terrors and sleepwalking, is not suggestive of emotional difficulties unless these difficulties are secondary to the wetting itself.

The incidence of enuresis decreases from about 15–18 percent at age 5 years to 2–5 percent after age 12 (Table 6.4) with about a 20 percent. spontaneous cure rate each year (McLain, 1979). The need for intervention depends on the age of the child, the frequency of wetting, and the effects the wetting has on patient and family. Occasional enuresis in a 5-year-old, for example, needs no treatment but careful explanation, whereas a 12-year-old who continues to void nightly may be suffering significantly even if the family is supportive.

The basic approach to the enuretic patient is a general evaluation (history, physical examination, and laboratory studies including urinalysis), explanation, and then, if intervention is important, usually behavioral trials and perhaps pharmacological measures. The general evaluation should be first to rule out organic factors such as urinary tract infection or abnormalities, diabetes, and neurological disorders including spina bifida or epilepsy. Then one should investigate features that suggest a benign condition, for example, a positive family history, the occurrence of wetting in the first one-

Table 6.4.   Prevalence of Nocturnal Bed Wetting in Males and Females by Age

Age (yr)	Boys (%)	Girls (%)
1–2	100	100
2–3	75	60
3–4	40	30
4–5	20	15
5–6	18	15
6–7	15	15
7–8	15	10
8–9	12	10
9–10	12	7
10–11	10	7
11–12	5	5
12 +	2–5	2–3

Reprinted by permission of the publisher, from Ferber and Rivinus (1979).

third of the night, and absence of any period six months or longer without any wetting (i.e., primary as opposed to secondary enuresis). Although true secondary enuresis may in fact be associated with a greater likelihood of organic disorder, enuresis may fluctuate, and a period of only relative dryness may be reported as "dry" by the family unless they are carefully questioned. Explanation and reassurance are vital to help alleviate feelings of shame and guilt.

Behavioral interventions include giving the child increased responsibility (Marshall, Marshall, and Lyon, 1973) and treating him in a more adult manner, emphasizing growing up rather than regressive tendencies. The child may take over, or at least help with, linen changing and he should not be in diapers. Use of a star chart (Marshall, Marshall, and Lyon, 1973) for younger children focuses attention on the dry days and can be quite helpful in certain cases. Bladder training exercises, in which the child holds his urine as long as possible at a certain time each day and then measures output trying to beat the previous mark, are based on the finding of decreased functional bladder capacities and increased urinary frequency in these patients. Good results have been reported (Starfield and Mellits, 1968). This method may be combined with use of a star chart. Close follow-up will help assure that advice is carried out, and review of star chart and volume records by the health care provider can have a great motivational influence on the child.

A behavioral method with an excellent reported cure rate is the so-called bell-and-pad (Behrle, Elkin, and Laybourne, 1956; Forsythe and Redmond, 1970), a device that rings an alarm when the patient wets. This presumably helps the patient learn to associate previously ignored prevoiding bladder sensations (even in sleep) with a need to generate arousal and voluntary bladder control. Although units are available in the United States, they have been used much more in Britain. Limiting fluids after dinner is reasonable if only because the volume of urine may be decreased, although the frequency of wetting is only rarely altered. Severe restrictions should be avoided. On the other hand, increasing fluids before bed is often tried as a method of "overlearning" to consolidate gains made after successful use of bladder-training or bell-and-pad approaches. "Lifting" the child, i.e., waking him to void before he wets in bed, is only occasionally helpful and then usually in a child who voids once per night at a predictable time. Lifting may lead to dry nights but does nothing to solve the underlying problem, i.e., wetting continues any nights the child is not taken to the bathroom. Leaving a light on in the bathroom, slippers by the bedside, and even having a carpet on the bathroom floor may help some early-morning enuretics.

The standard drug treatment today is imipramine, usually started at 1 mg per kilogram of body weight or less; the lowest possible effective dosage should be used. Although this medication clearly is effective (Kales et al, 1977; Pouissant and Ditman, 1965; Kardash, Hellman, and Werry, 1968), it is controversial whether the effect is by central or peripheral action. Peripherally it has an anticholinergic effect, and urinary retention is a known side effect when this drug is used for other purposes. Unlike its antidepressant action, which clearly is a central one, it is usually effective on day one in treating enuresis. Also in support of a peripheral action is the finding that there is little effect on the amount or depth of slow wave sleep (Kales et al, 1977). On the other hand, other anticholinergics such as atropine and propantheline seem much less effective (McLain, 1979) and scopolamine is no better than the placebo control (Korczyn and Kish, 1979). And imipramine, but not other anticholinergic agents that are only peripherally active, also has been useful in suppressing sleep terrors and sleepwalking, presumably (though not definitely) by central effects. Imipramine does, in fact, suppress REM sleep and if REM mechanisms were responsible at least for slow wave sleep arousals (as discussed above), then this is a possible central mechanism. Most likely, central and peripheral factors are involved.

Although medication may be useful, it must be remembered that the enuretic child is not at risk for self (physical)-injury and in this regard the disorder is mainly an annoyance. Reassurance and counseling to patient and family may be sufficient. But some families seem to cope poorly, and the child is chastized, punished, ridiculed, and made to feel guilty or abnormal. Even a family that seems to be supportive may not be completely so. There is usually some anger toward the child and this may be expressed subtly, for example, "You can have a new bed when the wetting stops." Even in the best of circumstances, nightly wetting represents a significant emotional stress on the child approaching adolescence, and if requests are made for help, full effort is indicated. If behavioral treatment is not successful, a medication trial is perhaps warranted. Even then, it makes sense to taper gradually about every three months, despite a high rate of relapse, to avoid unnecessary treatment. Also, once an effective dosage is ascertained, it may be used in specific instances to allow the child to attend summer camp, go on trips, or sleep at a friend's house. With this option available, wetting at other times may be better tolerated.

SUDDEN INFANT DEATH SYNDROME

Sudden infant death syndrome (SIDS) initially seems different from basically all other sleep disorders, since by definition it is characterized by a single symptom that has to occur at a certain age—death in infancy. This occurs most often during the usual sleep hours and hence is at least a disorder associated with sleep, a parasomnia. Some would suspect, however, that it would be best classified along with sleep apnea, but this remains to be definitely proved.

Current research into SIDS has been the topic of several recent reviews (Naeye, 1980; Valdés-Dapena, 1980; Hasselmeyer and Hunter, 1975; Read, Williams, Hensley, et al, 1979; Guntheroth, 1977). It does seem most likely that several factors are involved and hence the final cause of death could be different for different infants. In any case, SIDS remains the most common cause of infant mortality beyond the neonatal period. The rate of occurrence ranges from 0.67 to 6.56 per 1,000 live births depending on the particular patient population studied. The overall rate is most likely between 2 and 3 per 1,000 births. The highest incidence has been reported for American Indians. Other risk factors are summarized as follows:

1. Major risk factors
    Previous care in neonatal intensive care nursery
    Previous sibling(s) dying from SIDS
    Narcotic addiction in the mother during pregnancy
2. General or minor risk factors
    Low socioeconomic status
    Young maternal age
    Short interpregnancy interval
    Maternal smoking
    Prematurity
    Low birth weight
    Male sex

If SIDS is viewed as a sleep disorder with only one manifestation, death, then there is little hope to be able to identify patients ahead of time and prevent it. Recent research, however, suggests that patients at risk are physiologically different from those who are not and that autonomic nervous system function may in some way be impaired in these infants. Thus the infants may be suffering from a syndrome that is always present and for which death is a potential and extreme, rather than the only, manifestation. Many studies have been carried out on supposed near-miss infants (who may or may not have "almost" suffered SIDS) and some have shown increased numbers of mixed and obstructive apneas, especially at night (Guilleminault, Ariagno, Koroblein, et al, 1981), increased periodic breathing (Kelly and Shannon, 1979), alveolar hypoventilation (Shannon and Kelly, 1977), and altered ventilatory responses (Shannon and Kelly, 1978; Brady, Ariagno, Watts, et al, 1978). Smaller QT indices reported in one study (Haddad, Epstein, Epstein, et al, 1979) were not confirmed in another (Kelly, Shannon, and Liberthson, 1977). Pathological studies now suggest that repeated hypoxic events may have occurred over weeks and months before the terminal one (Naeye, 1980; Valdés-Dapena, 1980). Studies also suggest these physiological differences may be genetically determined. Subsequent siblings of SIDS victims are at increased risk (Froggatt, Lynas, and MacKenzie, 1971). In one study, siblings of SIDS victims were found to show increased periodic breathing (Kelly, Walker, Cahen, et al, 1980), whereas another group showed increased heart and respiratory rates but actually decreased respiratory pauses (Hoppenbrouwers, Hodgman, McGinty, et al,

1980; Harper, Leake, Hoppenbrouwers, et al, 1978). It has also been noted that parents of victims show decreased ventilatory responsiveness to carbon dioxide with and without increased airway resistance when compared with parents of controls (Schiffman, Westlake, Santiago, et al, 1980). Prospective studies have found higher incidences of subtle or not so subtle neurobehavioral abnormalities in patients who ultimately die (Anderson-Huntington and Rosenblith, 1976; Thomen, 1976). In addition, SIDS is more common in infants who are born prematurely, are of low birth weight, require special care as a newborn, and/or whose mother abused narcotics during pregnancy (Valdés-Dapena, 1980).

If respiratory obstruction is at fault, factors similar to those postulated for older children and adults may be important, such as posterior displacement of the tongue, relaxation of pharyngeal muscles, and altered control of the reflux airway. Nasal obstruction and obligate nose breathing (Swift and Emery, 1973; Steinschneider, 1975), airway obstruction secondary to neck flexion (Thach and Stark, 1979), or laryngospasm after gastroesophageal reflux are some of the other mechanisms that have been postulated. To date, evidence suggests that respiratory factors are responsible for the majority of deaths from SIDS, with nonrespiratory causes (for example, cardiac conduction abnormalities) (Keeton, Southall, Rutter, et al, 1978; Lipsitt, Starner, Oh, et al, 1979) accounting for a minority.

Treatment of previously resuscitated infants undergoing near-miss episodes or others considered to be at risk for whatever reason is still controversial. The use of home monitoring is being advocated and evaluated in a number of centers. This seems rational, may (or may not) be reassuring to parents, and ultimately may prove to be a necessary intervention, but selection of which patients to monitor and when to stop monitoring is difficult. Even when the alarm rings and the infant is resuscitated, it may be impossible to determine if the efforts were really necessary. Patients in whom the need is most clear-cut are those who have had several major near-miss episodes and in whom sleep studies show multiple long apneas. These children certainly cannot simply be sent home without monitoring and without teaching their parents cardiopulmonary resuscitation. Theophylline has been quite useful in helping to normalize respiratory patterns in some of these patients (Kelly and Shannon, 1981a,b). Atropine has been reported useful in cases of presumed recurrent laryngospasm (Kelly and Shannon, 1981a). Tracheostomies are seldom done but should be considered as future treatment if there is sufficient evidence of obstruction (Kelly and Shannon, 1981a,b).

HEAD BANGING (JACTATIO CAPITIS)

Head banging and head rolling as sleep disorders are both well recognized and poorly understood. They seem to occur in about 5 percent of normal children (Sallustro and Atwell, 1978; Kravitz, Rosenthal, Teplitz, et al,

1960; Kravitz and Boehm, 1971), although incidence figures from 3.3 percent (Levy and Patrick, 1928) to 15.2 percent (de Lissovoy, 1961, 1962) have been reported. Symptoms usually start by around age 9 months and abate by age 3 years; for head banging there is 3 to 1 male predominance. At times these rhythmic patterns may begin as early as 3 or 4 months of life. Rarely do they start later than early in the second year. Body rocking often starts by around 6 months, and rocking behavior frequently precedes the development of head banging (Lourie, 1949; Kravitz and Boehm, 1971; de Lissovoy, 1962). Head banging and body rocking are most commonly done on all fours, but other positions may be used as well (de Lissovoy, 1962). Episodes usually last less than 15 minutes, are most common in pre-sleep periods, and recur after nighttime awakenings apparently to aid the transition back to sleep. They may last only a few weeks or months or be more persistent. In any case, symptoms are usually gone within 18 months of their onset. Most such children seem emotionally and intellectually intact and have normal or advanced motor skills (Sallustro and Atwell, 1978). No specific intervention is usually necessary.

The symptoms may be more marked, with the child showing prolonged periods of head banging, forceful rocking, and body rolling for up to several hours even to the point of damage to crib and bruising of forehead. Significant head injuries, however, do not occur in otherwise normal children. Padding around the crib or headboard may be useful, but often it will only be pushed aside. Allowing a forceful head banger to sleep on a mattress in the middle of the floor may help, but the child may simply crawl to the wall and bang there. Occasionally, setting a metronome to beat at the same frequency as the head banging or even putting a loud-ticking alarm clock in the child's room may lead to reduction or even disappearance of symptoms (Lourie, 1949). Increased rhythmical activity during the day, including use of rocking chairs and time spent listening to music, is sometimes of apparent benefit.

Head banging may occur during full alertness as well as during sleep transition, and may be symptomatic of significant emotional disturbance (for example autism), emotional deprivation, sensory deprivation (blindness), and current family stresses. It may also represent learned attention-seeking behavior, in which case ignoring the symptom while providing adequate stimulation and attention at other times may lead to its decrease. Otherwise, full and careful evaluation is necessary and therapeutic intervention for the underlying emotional condition important.

Persistence of such behaviors beyond the toddler years is usually considered evidence of emotional problems, but this is not always so. Certainly, marked symptoms, for example, prolonged head banging or thrashing, is worrisome and probably has an emotional etiology; however, when such behavior occurs only in documented sleep (stages I and II), for example, as described in a two-year-old boy (Friedin, Jankowski, and Singer, 1979) and not as a sleep transition or waking behavior, this is less clear. This seems to be a physiological disorder of sleep that is not yet understood. Similarly, mild degrees of head or leg rolling in the presleep period (probably in waking and stage I) seem to have a physiological rather than emotional etiology in some older children, adolescents, and adults. One can speculate whether genetic factors are relevant, whether the symptoms represent learned habits that could be unlearned, or whether they represent automatic behaviors that are released in drowsiness and which possibly serve to aid (or even hinder) sleep transition. Pharmacological treatment of these disorders has not been satisfactory.

REFERENCES

Anders TF. Night waking in infants during the first year of life. Pediatrics 1979;63:860–64.

Anders TF, Carskadon MA, Dement WC. Sleep and sleepiness in children and adolescents. Pediatr Clin North Am 1980;27(1):29–43.

Anderson DR. Treatment of insomnia in a 13-year-old boy by relaxation training and reduction of parental attention. J Behav Ther Exp Psychiatry 1979;10:263–65.

Anderson-Huntington RB, Rosenblith JF. Central nervous system damage as a possible component of unexpected deaths in infancy. Dev Med Child Neurol 1976;18:480–92.

Arkin AM. Night-terrors as anomalous REM sleep component manifestation in slow-wave sleep. Waking Sleeping 1978;2:143–47.

Association of Sleep Disorders Centers. Diagnostic classification of sleep and arousal disorders. 1st ed. Prepared by the Sleep Disorders Classification Committee, Roffwarg HP, Chairman. Sleep 1979;2(1):1–137.

Bakwin H. The genetics of enuresis. In: Kolvin I, MacKeith RC, Meadow SR, eds. Bladder control and enuresis. Philadelphia: JB Lippincott, 1973:73–77.

Bax MCO. Sleep disturbance in the young child. Br Med J 1980;280:1177–79.

Beal VA. Termination of night feeding in infancy. J Pediatr 1969;75:690–92.

Behrle FC, Elkin MT, Laybourne PC. Evaluation of a conditioning device in the treatment of nocturnal enuresis. Pediatrics 1956;17:849–56.

Beitman BD, Carlin AS. Night terrors treated with imipramine. Am J Psychiatry 1979;136:1087–88.

Bernal J. Night waking in infancy during the first 14 months. Dev Med Child Neurol 1973;15:760–69.

Billiard M, Guilleminault WC, Dement WC. A menstruation-linked periodic hypersomnia. Neurology (Minneap) 1975;25:436–43.

Bland JW, Edwards FK, Brinsfield D. Pulmonary hypertension with congestive heart failure in childen with chronic upper airway obstruction. Am J Cardiol 1969;23:830–37.

Brady JP, Ariagno RL, Watts JL, Goldman SL, Dumpit FM. Apnea, hypoxemia, and aborted sudden infant death symdrome. Pediatrics 1978;62:686–91.

Broughton R. Sleep disorders: disorders of arousal? Science 1968;159:1070–78.

Broughton R, Gastaut H. Further polygraphic sleep studies of enuresis nocturna (intravesicular pressures). Electroencephalogr Clin Neurophysiol 1964;16:626.

Busby K, Firestone P, Pivik RT. Sleep patterns in hyperkinetic and normal children. Sleep 1981;4(4):366–83.

Carey W. Night waking and temperament in infancy. J Pediatr 1974;84:756–58.

Carskadon MA, Harvey K, Duke P, Anders TF, Litt IF, Dement WC. Pubertal changes in daytime sleepiness. Sleep 1980;2(4):453–60.

Czeisler CA, Richardson GS, Coleman R, Dement WC, Weitzman ED. Successful non-drug treatment of delayed sleep phase syndrome with chronotherapy: resetting a biological clock in man. Sleep Res 1979;8:178.

de Lissovoy V. Headbanging in early childhood. A study of incidence. J Pediatr 1961;58:803–5.

de Lissovoy V. Headbanging in early childhood. Child Dev 1962;33:43–56.

Dixon KN, Monroe LJ, Jakim S. Insomniac children. Sleep 1981;4(3):313–18.

Douglas J, Richman N. Sleep management manual. In-house publication, Department of Psychological Medicine, Great Ormond Street, Children's Hospital, London, 1982.

Easson WM. The early manifestations of adolescent thought disorder. J Clin Psychiatry 1979;2:469–76.

Elias MF, Nicolson N, Bora C, Johnston J. Effect of maternal care on social and emotional behavior of infants during the first year. Research report prepared for Society for Research in Child Development, Detroit, April 1983.

Feinberg I. Changes in sleep cycle patterns with age. J Psychiatr Res 1974;10:282–306.

Feinberg I, Hibi S, Brown M, Cavness C, Westerman G, Small A. Sleep amphetamine effects in MBDS and normal subjects. Arch Gen Psychiatry 1974;31:723–31.

Ferber R. Solve your child's sleep problem. New York: Simon & Schuster, 1985.

Ferber R, Boyle MP, Belfer M. Initial experience of a pediatric sleep disorders clinic. Sleep Res 1981a;10:194.

Ferber R, Boyle MP, Belfer M. "Insomnia" in toddlers seen in a pediatric sleep disorders clinic. Sleep Res 1981b;10:195.

Ferber R, Boyle MP. Confusional arousals in infants and toddlers (not quite pavor nocturnus). Sleep Res 1983a;12:241.

Ferber R, Boyle MP. Delayed sleep phase syndrome versus motivated sleep phase delay in adolescents. Sleep Res 1983b;12:239.

Ferber R, Boyle MP. Nocturnal fluid intake: a cause of, not treatment for, sleep disruption in infants and toddlers. Sleep Res 1983c;12:243.

Ferber R, Boyle MP. Phase shift dyssomnia in early childhood. Sleep Res 1983d;12:242.

Ferber R, Boyle MP. Sleeplessness in infants and toddlers: sleep initiation difficulty masquerading as a sleep maintenance insomnia. Sleep Res 1983e;12:240.

Ferber R, Friedman E, Dietz W. Obstructive sleep apnea in childhood: 80 cases. Sleep Res 1983;12:245.

Ferber R, Rivinus TM. Practical approaches to sleep disorders of childhood. Med Times 1979;107(6):71–80.

Ferber R, Rivinus TM. Sleep disorders in adolescence. Transitions 1980;3(5):12–14.

Fisher C, Kahn E, Edwards A, Davis DM. A psychophysiological study of nightmares and night terrors. I. Physiological aspects of the stage 4 night terror. J Nerv Ment Dis 1973a;157(2):75–98.

Fisher C, Kahn E, Edwards A, Davis DM. A psychophysiological study of night-mares and night terrors. II. The suppression of stage 4 night terrors with diazepam. Arch Gen Psychiatry 1973b;28:252–59.

Fisher C, Kahn E, Edwards A, Davis DM, Fine J. A psychophysiological study of nightmares and night terrors. III. Mental content and recall of stage 4 night terrors. J Nerv Ment Dis 1974;158(3):174–88.

Forsythe W, Redmond A. Enuresis and the electric alarm: study of 200 cases. Br Med J 1970;1:211–13.

Fraiberg S. On the sleep disturbances of early childhood. Psychoanal Stud Child 1950;5:285–309.

Friedin MR, Jankowski JJ, Singer WD. Nocturnal headbanging as a sleep disorder: a case report. Am J Psychiatry 1979;136:1469–70.

Froggatt P, Lynas MA, MacKenzie G. Epidemiology of sudden unexpected death in infants (cot death); report of a collaborative study in Northern Ireland. Ulster Med J 1971;40:116.

Fujita S, Zorick F, Conway W, Roth T, Hartse KM, Piccione PM. Uvulo-palato-pharyngoplasty: a new surgical treatment for upper airway sleep apnea. Sleep Res 1980;9:197.

Fujita S, Zorick F, Koshorek GJ, Wittig R, Conway W, Roth T. Treatment of upper airway sleep apnea with uvulo-palato-pharyngoplasty (UPP). Sleep Res 1981;10:197.

Fujita S, Conway W, Zorick F, Sicklesteel J, Roehrs T, Wittig R, Roth T. Evaluation of the effectiveness of uvulopalatopharyngoplasty. Abstract presented at the Fourth International Congress of Sleep Research, Bologna, July 1983.

Goodman RS, Goodman M, Gootman N, Cohen H. Cardiac and pulmonary failure secondary to adenotonsillar hypertrophy. Laryngoscope 1976;86:1367–74.

Guilleminault WC. The sleep apnea syndromes. Annu Rev Med 1976;27:465–84.

Guilleminault WC, Ariagno R, Korobkin R, Coons S, Owen-Boeddiker M, Baldwin R. Sleep parameters and respiratory variables in "near-miss" sudden infant death syndrome. Pediatrics 1981;68:354–60.

Guilleminault WC, Dement WC, eds. Sleep apnea syndromes. New York: Alan R. Liss, 1978.

Guilleminault WC, Eldridge FL, Simmons FB, Dement WC. Sleep apnea in eight children. Pediatrics 1976;58(1):23–30.

Guilleminault WC, Korobkin R, Winkle R. A review of 50 children with obstructive sleep apnea syndrome. Lung 1981;159:275–87.

Guntheroth WG. Sudden infant death syndrome (crib death). Am Heart J 1977;93(6):784–93.

Haddad GG, Epstein RA, Epstein MA, Leistner HL, Marino PA, Mellins RB. The QT interval in aborted sudden infant death syndrome infants. Pediatr Res 1979;13:136–38.

Haig JR, Schroeder CS, Schroeder SR. Effects of methylphenidate on hyperactive children's sleep. Psychopharmacology (Berlin) 1974;37:185–88.

Hallgren B. Nocturnal enuresis, aetiological aspects. Acta Paediatr Scand [Suppl] 1958;118:66–74.

Harper RM, Leake B, Hoppenbrouwers T, Sterman MB, McGinty DJ, Hodgman J. Polygraphic studies of normal infants and infants at risk for the sudden infant death syndrome: heart rate and variability as a function of state. Pediatr Res 1978;12:778–85.

Hasselmeyer EG, Hunter JC. The sudden infant death syndrome. Obstet Gynecol Annu 1975;4:213–36.

Hauri P. The sleep disorders. Kalamazoo, Mich.: Upjohn Scope Publications, 1977:22–34.

Hauri P. Biofeedback techniques in the treatment of chronic insomnia. In: Williams RL, Karacan I, eds. Sleep disorders, diagnosis and treatment. New York: John Wiley & Sons, 1978:145–59.

Hauri P. Behavioral treatment of insomnia. Med Times 1979;107(6):36–47.

Hauri P, Olmstead E. Childhood-onset insomnia. Sleep 1980;3(1):59–65.

Hertzman J. High school mental hygiene survey. Am J Orthopsychiatry 1948;18:238–56.

Hoppenbrouwers T, Hodgman JE, McGinty D, Harper RM, Sterman MB. Sudden infant death syndrome: sleep apnea and respiration in subsequent siblings. Pediatrics 1980;66:205–14.

Illingworth RS. Sleep problems in the first three years. Br Med J 1951;1:722–28.

Illingworth RS. Sleep problems of children. Clin Pediatr 1966;5:45–48.

Jones DPH, Verduyn CM. Behavioural management of sleep problems. Arch Dis Child 1983;58:442–4.

Kales A, Jacobson A, Paulson MJ, Kales JD, Walter RD. Somnabulism: psychophysiological correlates. I. All-night EEG studies. Arch Gen Psychiatry 1966;14:586–94.

Kales A, Kales JD, Jacobson A, Humphrey FJ, Soldatos CR. Effects of imipramine on enuretic frequency and sleep stages. Pediatrics 1977;60:431–36.

Kales A, Soldatos CR, Caldwell AB, et al. Somnabulism: clinical characteristics and personality patterns. Arch Gen Psychiatry 1980;37:1406–10.

Kales JD, Jacobson A, Kales A. Sleep disorders in children. In: Abt L, Riess BF, eds. Progress in clinical psychology. New York: Grune & Stratton, 1969:63–75.

Kales JD, Soldatos CR, Caldwell AB, Charney DS, Martin ED. Night terrors: clinical characteristics and personality patterns. Arch Gen Psychiatry 1980;37:1413–17.

Kales JD, Kales A, Soldatos CR, Chamberlin K, Martin ED. Sleep walking and night terrors related to a febrile illness. Am J Psychiatry 1979;136(9):1214–15.

Karacan I, Anch M, Thornby JI, Okawa M, Williams RL. Longitudinal sleep patterns during pubertal growth: four-year follow-up. Pediatr Res 1975;9:842–46.

Karacan I, Wolff SM, Williams RL, et al. The effects of fever on sleep and dream patterns. Psychosomatics 1968;9:331–39.

Kardash S, Hellman E, Werry J. Efficacy of imipramine in childhood enuresis: a double-blind control study with placebo. Can Med Assoc J 1968;99:263–66.

Keeton BR, Southall E, Rutter N, Anderson RH, Shinebourne EA, Southall DP. Cardiac conduction disorders in six infants with "near miss" sudden infant deaths. Br Med J 1978;2:600–1.

Kelly DH, Shannon DC. Periodic breathing in infants with near-miss sudden infant death syndrome. Pediatrics 1979;63:355–60.

Kelly DH, Shannon DC. Episodic complete airway occlusion in infants. Pediatrics 1981a;67:823–27.

Kelly DH, Shannon DC. Treatment of apnea and excessive periodic breathing in the full-term infant. Pediatrics 1981b;68:183–86.

Kelly DH, Shannon DC, Liberthson RR. The role of the QT interval in the SIDS. Circulation 1977;55:633–35.

Kelly DH, Walker AM, Cahen L, Shannon DC. Periodic breathing in siblings of sudden infant death syndrome victims. Pediatrics 1980;66:515–20.

Kessler S. Genetic factors in narcolepsy. In: Guilleminault WC, Dement WC, Passouant P, eds. Narcolepsy. New York: Spectrum, 1976:285–302.

Khan A, Rechtschaffen A. Sleep patterns and sleep spindles in hyperkinetic children. Sleep Res 1978;7:137.

Kleitman N. Mental hygiene of sleep in children. Nerv Child 1949;8(1):63–66.

Korczyn AD, Kish I. The mechanism of imipramine in enuresis nocturna. Clin Exp Pharmacol Physiol 1979;6:31–35.

Korlath HJ, Baizerman M, Williams S. Twin city adolescent health attitudes, knowledge, and behavior. Center Q Focus 1976; 1–6.

Kravath RE, Pollak CP, Borowiecki B. Hypoventilation during sleep in children who have lymphoid airway obstruction treated by nasopharyngeal tube and tonsillectomy and adenoidectomy. Pediatrics 1977;59(6):865–71.

Kravath RE, Pollak CP, Borowiecki B, Weitzman ED. Obstructive sleep apnea and death associated with surgical correction of velopharyngeal incompetence. J Pediatr 1980;96(4):645–48.

Kravitz H, Boehm JJ. Rhythmic habit patterns in infancy: their sequence, age of onset, and frequency. Child Dev 1971;42:399–413.

Kravitz H, Rosenthal V, Teplitz Z, Murphy JB, Lesser RE. A study of head-banging in infants and children. Dis Nerv Syst 1960;21:203–8.

Levin M. Periodic somnolence and morbid hunger: a new syndrome. Brain 1936;59:494–515.

Levy AM, Tabakin BS, Harrison JS, Narkewicz RM. Hypertrophied adenoids causing pulmonary hypertension and severe congestive failure. N Engl J Med 1967;277:506–11.

Levy DM, Patrick HT. Relation of infantile convulsions, headbanging, and breath-holding to fainting and headaches (migraine?) in the parents. Arch Neurol Psychiatry 1928;19:865–87.

Lipsitt LP, Starner WQ, Oh W, Barrett J, Truex RC. Wolff-Parkinson-White and sudden infant death syndromes. Letter to the editor. N Engl J Med 1979;300:1111.

Logan DG. Antidepressant treatment of recurrent anxiety attacks and night terrors. Ohio State Med J 1979;75:653–55.

Lourie RS. The role of rhythmic patterns in childhood. Am J Psychiatry 1949;105:653–60.

Lugaresi E, Coccagna G, Mantovani M. Hypersomnia with periodic apneas. New York: Spectrum, 1978.

Luisada PV. REM deprivation and hyperactivity in children. Chicago Med School Q 1969;28:97–108.

Luke MJ, Mehrizi A, Folger GM, Rowe D. Chronic nasopharyngeal obstruction as a cause of cardiomegaly, cor pulmonale and pulmonary edema. Pediatrics 1966;37:762–68.

Mangot D, Orr WC, Smith RO. Sleep apnea, hypersomnolence, and upper airway obstruction secondary to adenotonsillar enlargement. Arch Otolaryngol 1977;103(7):383–86.

Marks PA, Monroe LJ. Correlates of adolescent poor sleepers. J Abnorm Psychol 1976;85:243–46.

Marshall S, Marshall H, Lyon R. Enuresis: an analysis of various therapeutic approaches. Pediatrics 1973;52:813–17.

Massumi RA, Sarin RK, Pooya M, et al. Tonsillar hypertrophy, airway obstruction, alveolar hypoventilation and cor pulmonale in twin brothers. Dis Chest 1969;55:110–14.

McLain LG. Childhood enuresis. Curr Probl Pediatr 1979;9(8):2–36.

Menashe VD, Fearron C, Miller M. Hypoventilation and cor pulmonale due to chronic upper airway obstruction. J Pediatr 1965;67:198–203.

Moore T, Ucko LE. Nightwaking in early infancy. Part 1. Arch Dis Child 1957;32:333–42.

Naeye RL. Sudden infant death. Sci Am 1980;242(4):56–62.

Navelet Y, Anders T, Guilleminault WC. Narcolepsy in children. In: Guilleminault WC, Dement WC, Passouant P, eds. Narcolepsy. New York: Spectrum, 1976:171–77.

Noonan JA. Reversible cor pulmonale due to hypertrophied tonsils and adenoids. Studies in two cases. Circulation 1965;32(Suppl 2):164.

Oswald I. Sleep research and mental illness. Psychol Med 1975;5:1–3.

Pesikoff RB, Davis PC. Treatment of pavor nocturnus and somnabulism in children. Am J Psychiatry 1971;128:134–37.

Phillipson EA. Breathing disorders during sleep. Basics of respiratory physiology. 1979;7(3):1–6.

Pierce CM. Dream studies in enuresis research. Can Psychiatr Assoc J 1963;8:415–19.

Pierce CM, Whitman RM, Maas JW, Gay ML. Enuresis and dreaming. Arch Gen Psychiatry 1961;4:166.

Pouissant AF, Ditman KS. A controlled study of imipramine (Tofranil) in the treatment of childhood enuresis. J Pediatr 1965;67:283–90.

Preston MI. Late behavioral aspects found in cases of prenatal, natal, and postnatal anoxia. J Pediatr 1945;26:353–66.

Price VA, Coates TJ, Thoresen CE, Grinstead OA. Prevalence and correlates of poor sleep among adolescents. Am J Dis Child 1978;132:583–86.

Ragins N, Schachter S. A study of sleep behavior in two-year-old children. J Am Acad Child Psychiatry 1971;10:464–80.

Rapoport DM, Sorkin B, Garay SM, Goldring RM. Reversal of the "pickwickian syndrome" by long-term use of nocturnal nasal-airway pressure. N Engl J Med 1982;307:931–3.

Read DJC, Williams AL, Hensley W, Edwards M, Beal S. Sudden infant deaths: some current research strategies. Med J Aust 1979;2:236–44.

Richman N. A community survey of characteristics of one- to two-year-olds with sleep disruptions. J Am Acad Child Psychiatry 1981;20(2):281–91.

Roberts KE, Schoellkopf JA. Eating, sleeping, and elimination practices of a group of two-and-one-half-year-old children. Am J Dis Child 1951;82:121–52.

Saint-Laurent J, Batini C, Broughton R, Gastaut H. Etude polygraphique de l'énurésis nocturne chez l'enfant épileptique. Rev Neurol (Paris) 1963;108:106.

Sallustro F, Atwell CW. Body rocking, headbanging, and head rolling in normal children. J Pediatr 1978;93:704–8.

Schiffman PL, Westlake RE, Santiago TV, Edelman NH. Ventilatory control in parents of victims of sudden-infant-death syndrome. N Engl J Med 1980;302:486–91.

Silvestri R, Guilleminault C, Simmons FB. Palato-pharyngo-plasty (PPP), the Stanford experience. Sleep Res 1982;11:175.

Shannon DC, Kelly D. Impaired regulation of alveolar ventilation and the sudden infant death syndrome. Science 1977;197:367–68.

Shannon DC, Kelly D. Abnormal ventilatory responses to CO_2 during quiet sleep in aborted SIDS. Chest 1978;73(2 Suppl):301.

Shepherd F. Disturbed sleep in infancy and childhood. Hatfield, England, 1948.

Sours J, Frumkin P, Indermill R. Somnabulism: its clinical significance and dynamic meaning in late adolescence and adulthood. Arch Gen Psychiatry 1963;9:400–13.

Starfield B. Functional bladder capacity in enuretic and nonenuretic children. J Pediatr 1967;70:777–81.

Starfield B, Mellits ED. Increase in functional bladder capacity and improvement in enuresis. J Pediatr 1968;72:483–87.

Steinschneider A. Nasopharyngitis and prolonged sleep apnea. Pediatrics 1975;56:967–71.

Sullivan CE, Issa FG, Berthon-Jones M, Eves L. Reversal of obstructive sleep apnoea by continuous positive airway pressure applied through the nares. Lancet 1981;1:862–5.

Swift PG, Emery JL. Clinical observations on response to nasal occlusion in infancy. Arch Dis Child 1973;48:947–51.

Talbot AR, Robertson LW. Cardiac failure with tonsil and adenoid hypertrophy. Arch Otolaryngol 1973;98:277–81.

Thach BT, Stark AR. Spontaneous neck flexion and airway obstruction during apneic spells in preterm infants. J Pediatr 1979;94:275–81.

Thomen E. Earliest behavioral developments of an infant who died of SIDS. In: Hasselmeyer EG, ed. Research perspectives in the sudden infant death syndrome. DHEW publ. no. (NIH) 76-1976. Washington, D.C.: National Institutes of Health, 1976.

Valdés-Dapena MA. Sudden infant death syndrome: a review of the medical literature 1974–1979. Pediatrics 1980;66:597–614.

Vullaimy D. The day and night output of urine in enuresis. Arch Dis Child 1956;31:439–43.

Webb W, Agnew H. Are we chronically sleep-deprived? Bull Psychosom Soc 1975;6:47–48.

Weil G, Goldfried MR. Treatment of insomnia in an eleven-year-old child through self-relaxation. Behav Ther 1973;4:282–94.

Weitzman ED, Czeisler CA, Coleman RM, Spielman AJ, Zimmerman JC, Dement WC. Delayed sleep phase syndrome. Arch Gen Psychiatry 1981;38:737–46.

Weitzman ED, Czeisler CA, Zimmerman JC, Ronda JM. Timing of REM and stages 3 and 4 sleep during temporal isolation in man. Sleep 1980;2(4)391–407.

Werry JS. Enuresis, a psychosomatic entity? Can Med Assoc J 1967;97:319–27.

Williams RL, Karacan I, Davis G. Sleep patterns of pubertal males. Pediatr Res 1972;6:643–47.

Williams RL, Karacan I, Hursch CJ. EEG of human sleep. New York: John Wiley & Sons, 1974.

CHAPTER 7

Sleep Pathophysiology in Medicine and Surgery
William C. Orr

Perhaps no area of human physiology has greater impact on the range of medical practice than the basic physiology of sleep. The choice of a particular specialty or subspecialty dictates that medical problems related to other organ systems are rarely encountered. The cardiologist would rarely deal with problems related to dysmenorrhea. Similarly, the gynecologist would generally not feel competent to deal appropriately with persistent complaints of chest pain. Both cardiologists and gynecologists, however, commonly encounter complaints of disordered sleep as well as the manifestations of sleep pathophysiology. For example, it is well known that cardiovascular and gonadal hormonal regulation are altered during sleep. Considering medical practice in general, there would seem to be no group more commonly presented with sleep complaints than the family practitioner and general internist. Thus knowledge of a practical approach to the patient with sleep complaints, as well as how altered sleep physiology can result in medical complications, would certainly enhance the patient care skills of every physician.

The difficulty and complexity of dealing with sleep pathophysiology in the clinical arena stems from the facts that sleep is a distinctly covert phenomenon rarely observed by the physician; altered physiology in the waking state does not necessarily suggest sleep pathology in any obvious fashion; and sleep complaints themselves often obscure the true underlying sleep pathology. Complaints of insomnia and excessive daytime sleepiness can be related to a potentially lethal sleep-related breathing disorder such as obstructive sleep apnea, or either complaint could be related to a purely functional disorder such as anxiety and/or depression. Dealing with the complaint itself is frequently frustrating and unproductive for the physician who does not have the capability of studying the patient during sleep.

The issues of diagnosis and management are further complicated by the obvious fact that sleeping behavior affects waking behavior and waking behavior affects sleeping behavior. This fact transcends every discipline of medicine, and once again emphasizes the importance of understanding sleep

159

pathophysiology. Integration of the fields of sleep physiology and clinical medicine has been facilitated and stimulated by the development of laboratory facilities to study objectively the physiology of sleep. With evaluation during sleep, the link between sleep pathophysiology and a variety of medical entities has been solidly established.

Clinical sleep facilities have been proliferating, and knowledge concerning the relationships between sleep physiology and a variety of medical specialties and subspecialties has been accumulating at a rapid pace. As a result of this remarkable growth, codification of this information has recently been published as a nosology of sleep disorders (Association of Sleep Disorders Centers, 1979). This chapter deals specifically with pathophysiological phenomena during sleep that produce and/or exacerbate a variety of medical conditions. Focus is on events that do not necessarily produce a clinical complaint concerning sleep. An example would be the altered nocturnal penile tumescence (NPT) in impotence secondary to diabetes. Alterations of sleep patterns after surgery and traumatic head injury and their prognostic value are discussed. Also examined are the effects of commonly used medications on sleep patterns, and the complications of sleep-related gastroesophageal reflux (GER).

COMMONLY USED DRUGS AND SLEEP

The administration of drugs is as inherent to the practice of medicine as the history and physical examination. Consideration of the appropriate pharmacological treatment of any condition involves an assessment of the potential benefit and side effects of the medication. The effects of a hypnotic medication on physiological sleep patterns provide data concerning both the beneficial and noxious effects of the compound. Certain psychotropic drugs, for example, tricyclic antidepressants, have a rather profound impact on sleep patterns, which of course, would have to be considered a side effect. Although little attention has been given to the direct or indirect effects of other commonly used medications on sleep patterns and nocturnal physiology, over the last 10 years literally hundreds of studies have been done on various psychotropic compounds (see Kay, Blackburn, Buckingham, et al, 1976, for a comprehensive review) (1) because of an inherent belief that alterations in the endogenous sleep pattern would produce marked alterations on waking behavior; and (2) in an attempt to provide a useful bioassay of drug effects.

There are few if any well-controlled studies that would suggest that an alteration—for example, the amount of rapid eye movement (REM) or nonrapid eye movement (NREM) sleep—in the intrinsic sleep pattern has, in and of itself, any obvious deleterious effect. Reduction in sleep onset latency, the number of awakenings, subjective responses, and subsequent performance would appear to be more clinically useful criteria by which to evaluate the efficacy of a hypnotic drug (Kagan, Harwood, Rickels, et al, 1975). Numerous studies have demonstrated that some of these agents produce subsequent deficits in performance and memory (Johnson and Chernik, 1981).

Altered drug metabolism has been described in the elderly, rendering this patient population considerably more susceptible to the toxic effects of any drug (Williamson, 1980). This is especially noteworthy for clinicians since it is well established that sleep complaints and hypnotic drug use are appreciably more common among the elderly (Miles and Dement, 1980). Thus hypnotic drugs with reputed minimal side effects may induce psychotic-like symptoms when used in a geriatric population (Miles and Dement, 1980).

Hypnotics

The effects of hypnotic drugs on sleep patterns appear to be relatively similar despite structural differences among the barbiturates, benzodiazepines, and nonbarbiturate hypnotics. Most of these compounds will suppress REM sleep and produce minimal but variable effects on NREM sleep. Most result in increases in spindling activity and mildly suppressed slow wave sleep. As suggested above and pointed out in a detailed review of the effects of hypnotic drugs on sleep patterns by Freemon (1975), the clinical significance of these findings remains unclear. A consensus appears to be developing that these alterations, unless egregious, probably have little clinical significance. Thus in evaluating the efficacy of hypnotic drugs, effects of variables such as sleep-onset latency and awakenings, subjective improvement in sleep (through patient reports), and subsequent decrements (or improvements) in performance would appear to be the most clinically important.

There appears to be little to choose from between barbiturates and benzodiazepine hypnotics in terms of alterations in sleep patterns, reductions in latency of sleep onset, and awakenings after sleep onset. The benzodiazepines clearly have advantages in terms of their margin of safety, tolerance development, and withdrawal effects (Kay et al, 1976). In addition, virtually all hypnotic drugs in sufficient dosages will produce performance decrements. Further complicating this issue is the fact that there appears to be little in the way of a discernible monotonic relationship between the half-life of these compounds and their physiological and behavioral effects (Johnson and Chernik, 1981).

The perfect hypnotic has been characterized as a compound that "should promote sleep quickly, alter the architecture and patterns of sleep only toward the norm, be satisfactorily deactivated by morning awakening, influence no other body system or drug action, have a wide margin of safety, and be reliably effective without danger of tolerance or dependence" (Orr,

Altshuler, and Stahl, 1982). Obviously, no such medication exists and the physician must therefore choose the agent that most closely approaches the ideal. As has been noted, in selecting a hypnotic drug, less emphasis should be placed on the degree to which the compound alters sleep architecture and more on its subsequent effects on behavior. A discussion of the appropriate use of hypnotics, designed specifically for the practicing physician, is available in a recently published book (Orr, Altshuler, and Stahl, 1982).

Other important but less well investigated phenomena include the effects of hypnotics on nocturnal physiology. For example, it is becoming increasingly obvious that respiratory functioning is compromised even in healthy persons during sleep. The delicate balance of normal respiratory physiology can be affected by drugs that depress the central nervous system, resulting in a potentially dangerous situation in some patients. Recent studies have documented an exacerbation of upper airway obstructive episodes during sleep with administration of hypnotic drugs in the elderly and in patients with chronic obstructive pulmonary disease (Coburn, Zeiger, Guilleminault, et al, 1982; Guilleminault and Silvestri, 1982). Increased episodes of obstructive sleep apnea have recently been shown to be provoked by alcohol ingestion, with a mild to moderate incidence of airway obstruction during sleep (Scrima, Broudy, Nay, et al, 1982). Although further work needs to be done in this area, it suggests that individuals with a history of loud snoring with anecdotal observations of apnea should be administered hypnotic drugs only with the greatest caution. A documented history of obstructive sleep apnea would be a clear contraindication for the administration of hypnotics.

A particularly difficult problem in this area is management of the patient who has been taking hypnotic drugs chronically. Withdrawal presents a difficult and complex problem. Depending on the agent and the duration of use, the patient may experience the rebound of REM sleep to supranormal levels, and the associated fragmented and subjectively poor sleep that often accompanies hypnotic withdrawal (Freemon, 1975). These phenomena collectively result in a syndrome called rebound insomnia. It should be noted that studies to date suggest that this condition may be somewhat less likely to occur with certain benzodiazepine compounds (Kay et al, 1976).

Nevertheless, the prudent physician should realize that difficulties can be encountered with hypnotic withdrawal that create problems clinically in that the patient suddenly experiences the following sequence: (1) hypnotic withdrawal, (2) exacerbation of the insomnia problem, and (3) resumption of the hypnotic drug. Clinical experience has shown that after going several nights without the drug, this acute exacerbation resolves and the patient begins to sleep considerably better, or at least no worse than when taking the drug. It is the acute insomnia that is particularly difficult to manage because patients become uncomfortable and anxious, and they must be assured that this condition is temporary and that relief will be obtained in a few days. It may require nearly daily contact to nurture the patient through this situation. Rebound insomnia may occur in spite of very gradual reduction in dosage as recommended by Kales and associates (1974) by one therapeutic dose per week. If the physician adheres to this protocol, appropriately counsels the patient to expect this acute exacerbation, and follows this up with appropriate supportive measures, withdrawal from these agents can be effectively accomplished.

Antidepressant Drugs

Depression remains perhaps the most common psychiatric affliction, and over the last 15 to 20 years the development of pharmacological agents in its treatment remains a major accomplishment. The tricyclic antidepressants are currently recognized as the treatment of choice, particularly in cases of endogenous depression. These drugs are commonly used by psychiatrists and internists and are known to have profound effects on physiological sleep patterns (reviewed by both Kay et al, 1976, and Freemon, 1975). Most commonly noted are substantial REM sleep suppression and withdrawal REM rebound.

The effects of antidepressants on REM sleep are of considerable theoretical and some practical concern. Characteristic alterations have been described in endogenously depressed patients (Coble, Foster, and Kupfer, 1976; Kupfer, Foster, Reich, et al, 1976), including a decrease in latency of REM onset (the time from sleep onset to the first REM period), an increase in the density of eye movements during REM sleep, and decreases in the total percentage of REM sleep. Gillin et al (1979) confirmed these findings and suggested that polysomnographic patterns can accurately distinguish depressed and insomniac patients from normal persons. Kupfer and coworkers (1981) showed that the alterations in REM sleep values can predict the clinical response to tricyclic antidepressant medication. They found that a decrease in sleep onset latency and prolongation of REM onset latency predicted successful clinical response to amitriptyline therapy. Gillin et al (1978) demonstrated that patients who experienced appreciable clinical improvement while taking amitriptyline showed REM rebound subsequent to withdrawal of the medication.

These studies suggest some relationship between the neurobiology of REM sleep and the pathogenesis of depression. Vogel (1975) described considerable clinical improvement in patients with endogenous depression who underwent chronic REM deprivation in the sleep laboratory. He suggested that the short REM onset latency and the REM rebound encountered subsequent to withdrawal of REM-suppressing antidepressant medication is consistent with a "REM pressure" that is present in endogenous depression. Vogel hypothesizes that this state is associated with altered central neuron activity, which plays a major role in the pathogenesis of depression.

Studies concerned with the basic physiology and pharmacology of sleep have contributed greatly not only to our understanding of an important affective disorder, but also to more effective treatment of this condition.

Tryptophan

Numerous commonly ingested food constituents such as tryptophan and caffeine as well as alcohol have been shown to have appreciable effects on sleep. A series of investigations on tryptophan by Hartmann (1977) showed that, in sufficiently high doses (1 gm or more), tryptophan will reduce sleep onset latency. Hartmann and Spinwebber (1979) have further indicated that amounts less than 1 gm, although not producing statistically significant effects, will also reduce sleep onset latency in individuals with documented prolonged sleep onset latencies. Although the effects for 0.25 and 0.5 gm were marginal, the reduction in sleep onset latency with 1 gm was statistically significant. The authors attributed considerable clinical significance to this effect since they stated that the normal daily dietary intake of tryptophan ranges between 0.5 and 2 gm.

Unfortunately, the increasing awareness of the complexity of the relationship between dietary intake, peripheral and central metabolism of protein and carbohydrates, and their ultimate effect on sleep patterns is such that the study by Hartmann and Spinwebber is, at best, only suggestive. Other dietary constituents such as carbohydrates have also been shown to affect sleep patterns, and the brain uptake of tryptophan is affected not only by dietary intake of this amino acid, but by the relative concentration of protein and carbohydrates in the diet (Greenwood, Lader, Kantameneni, et al, 1975; Wurtman and Fernstrom, 1974). It has been demonstrated, for example, that a high-carbohydrate meal will facilitate brain uptake of tryptophan through the action of insulin, whereas a high-protein diet will elevate the serum but not the brain level of tryptophan.

An example of how failure to control these variables can mitigate the impact of an otherwise well-controlled study is shown in an experiment published by Al-Marashi and Freemon (1977). These investigators carefully controlled the dietary intake of tryptophan and studied four healthy control subjects given high- and low-tryptophan diets. They demonstrated that, in contrast to the Hartmann and Spinwebber study cited above, there was no alteration in sleep onset latency. They did, however, document a statistically significant reduction in awakenings after sleep onset and wake time after sleep onset with the high-tryptophan diet. The difficulties with a study such as this are reflected in the fact that the high-tryptophan diet was also high in protein compared to the low-tryptophan diet, and the low-tryptophan diet was much higher in carbohydrate content than the high-tryptophan diet. This creates other confounding variables and renders interpretation of this study nearly impossible in terms of the effect of dietary tryptophan on the sleep measurements reported. The main uncontrolled variables would be the content of carbohydrate, which has been shown to alter the uptake of brain tryptophan, and of protein, which delays uptake of tryptophan from the intestine due to competition from other amino acids.

Thus it could easily be argued that although the investigators produced a diet high in tryptophan content, by including a high concentration of protein and relatively low concentration of carbohydrate, there was a delayed increase in serum tryptophan concentration with little alteration in brain concentration of tryptophan as a result. On the other hand, since the low-tryptophan diet contained approximately twice the amount of carbohydrate, the actual brain uptake of tryptophan would be greatly facilitated, rendering the true brain concentration of tryptophan in these two conditions an imponderable. Perhaps the most carefully controlled and definitive study available at the present time was performed by Adam and Oswald (1979), in which both the amount of tryptophan and concentration of dietary carbohydrate were controlled. These investigators found no significant effects of tryptophan on sleep onset latency whether it was combined with high or low intake of dietary carbohydrate.

Caffeine

Another commonly ingested food that has been shown to have a considerable effect on physiological sleep patterns is caffeine. It has been studied most thoroughly by Karacan et al (1976), who demonstrated that a single cup of coffee prior to bedtime has no effect on sleep patterns. Two and four cups of coffee, however, and the equivalent amount of caffeine, in the same subjects produced significant increases in sleep onset latency and reductions in total sleep time. They noted only trivial alterations from the baseline data with decaffeinated coffee. Also of interest is the fact that subjective reports were coincident with objective sleep laboratory data. Similar alterations in sleep patterns have been documented in older subjects (mean age, 56 years) by Brezinova (1974). Total sleep time was decreased on the average by two hours, and the mean sleep onset latency was significantly prolonged. In view of the ubiquity of caffeine in such commonly ingested foods as cola drinks, coffee, and chocolate, the clinical relevance of these data is apparent.

Alcohol

Perhaps the most commonly used nonprescription hypnotic in our culture is alcohol, undoubtedly because of its known sedative properties. Sleep laboratory studies have shown, however, that this sedating effect is short lived (Rundell, Lester, Griffiths, et al, 1972). Awakenings are decreased during the first half of the night but increased toward the end of the sleeping interval. In addition, REM sleep is decreased, particularly in the first half of the night, and there is a REM rebound effect that is particularly notice-able in chronic alcoholics (Lester, Rundell, Cowden, et al, 1973). Certainly one of the most important considerations with regard to the effects of al-cohol relates to its synergistic effect with other medications such as hypnotics and other psychotropic compounds. Quite obviously, from the above com-ments concerning the central nervous system and respiratory depressant effects of hypnotic drugs and their demonstrated effect on sleep-related breathing disorders, synergistic effects that would undoubtedly exist with alcohol could be potentially fatal in susceptible individuals.

SLEEP PATTERNS FOLLOWING HEAD TRAUMA AND SURGERY

Alterations in the normal sleep pattern have been ascribed to certain en-dogenous and exogenous stresses. The normal endogenous sleep rhythm is felt to be a sensitive indicator of general cerebral functioning. As with the sedimentation rate, disruptions of this system are highly nonspecific, but they do suggest abnormal functioning. These alterations in normal sleep patterns can be of some clinical utility. This section focuses on the sleep patterns in comatose patients and those who have undergone surgical pro-cedures.

Coma

It is not surprising that a blow to the head resulting in a severe disturbance of consciousness would be sufficiently disruptive of general cerebral func-tioning to produce an alteration in sleep patterns. The normal expression of the REM and NREM cycles requires the fundamental integrity of the brainstem, diencephalon, and telencephalon. Chartrian, White, and Daly (1963) reported that in 11 patients who sustained traumatic head injuries followed immediately by coma, the presence of "sleeplike patterns" on elec-troencephalogram (EEG) were associated with a favorable outcome. A somewhat more detailed study related the presence of polygraphic sleep patterns more precisely to the patient's clinical status (Bergamasco, Ber-gamini, Doriguzzi, et al, 1968). In their group of 18 patients posttrauma there was a clear relationship between recovery from coma and the presence of typical polygraphical sleep patterns. In another study of eight patients with recent head trauma, a relationship was described between the cyclic organization of the sleep pattern and improvement in state of consciousness (Passouant, Cadilhac, Delange, et al, 1965).

Other studies have suggested that stages III and IV of NREM sleep are somewhat more sensitive to the effects of traumatic head injury (Jouvet, Pellin, and Mounier, 1962; Lenard and Pennigstorff, 1970). The study by

Jouvet and colleagues indicated that diffuse injury of the neocortex tends to abolish stages III and IV sleep while leaving the manifestations of REM reasonably well intact. They also pointed out that in cases of reversible disturbance of consciousness with both cortex and brainstem intact, both slow wave sleep and REM sleep tend to cycle in a normal fashion. Lenard and Penningstorff (1970) pointed out that since the structures of the midbrain and brainstem are the most susceptible to traumatic head injury and are intimately involved in the regulation of sleep, it is not surprising that there is considerable disruption of sleep patterns subsequent to traumatic head injury. Their study confirms the findings of the Jouvet group by showing that reductions in stages III and IV NREM sleep were somewhat more likely to occur with traumatic head injury in children. They also noted that some residual functional disturbances may persist even though symptoms have disappeared and the EEG appears normal. To effect optimal management of these patients, they emphasized a dynamic approach to the use of the clinical electroencephalogram that includes consideration of the characteristics of sleep. Collectively, these studies suggest the clinical utility of polygraphic sleep patterns and incorporation of basic sleep physiology into the management of patients following head injury. The rationale for this approach is cogently stated by Bergamasco et al (1968):

> It may be said that, the brain, without its facility of maintaining state of vigilance, can still keep a differentiated sleep wakefulness rhythm, its functional integrity can, in a broad sense, be presumed. The *presence of a differentiated rhythm,* then . . . allows us to *predict a possible recovery* of the highest functional expression of the brain, mainly the regulation of the conscious state [italics added; p. 377].

Following Surgical Procedures

Several studies have described profound subjective sleep disturbances following open-heart surgery that have been linked inferentially to the relatively high incidence of postoperative psychosis in this patient group (Egerton and Kay, 1964; Heller, Frank, Malm, et al, 1970). None of these studies, however, polygraphically documented either acute or chronic changes in sleep patterns in these patients. A study was undertaken in our laboratory to document acute and chronic (four to six weeks postoperative) disturbances in sleep patterns in patients undergoing open-heart surgery and a control group of patients undergoing a chest procedure without cardiopulmonary bypass. The data from this study documented long-term alterations (up to five to six weeks postoperatively) in both REM and NREM sleep following open-heart surgery. Patients undergoing a chest procedure without cardiopulmonary bypass (pneumonectomy) showed much more rapid recovery of normal sleep (Orr and Stahl, 1977).

Although it seemed clear from these data that patients undergoing thoracotomy alone appeared to recover normal sleep patterns (i.e., spindle sleep and REM) sooner, it seemed equally clear that the longer operative times involved in open-heart surgery played a significant role in the persistence of disturbed sleep patterns. More recently, Kavey and Altshuler (1979) studied sleep patterns in patients who had undergone a somewhat less traumatic surgical procedure, for example, herniorrhaphy. Although this study did not include postoperative follow-up beyond the initial hospitalization, their results very much resembled those of the thoracotomy group in the open-heart study discussed above. That is, there was profound acute suppression of both REM and stages III and IV sleep followed by a daily linear increase to near preoperative levels. In contrast to the open-heart surgical study, some REM rebound was noted in patients following herniorrhaphy. It is not clear to what extent this may have been secondary to REM suppression induced by postoperative administration of the analgesic meperidine. The REM suppression noted following open-heart procedures persisted into the four- to six-week follow-up studies, suggesting a more profound alteration in brain metabolic processes in this group. It is of interest in the herniorrhaphy study that patients' subjective reports of their sleep had little bearing on objective documentation of sleep patterns. Kavey and Altshuler emphasized that perfunctory inquiries concerning sleep were most unlikely to reveal significant results. The clinician would therefore do well to inquire in more detail concerning number of arousals, sleep onset latency, and early morning awakenings.

It would appear from this brief review that an awareness of altered sleep patterns subsequent to physical trauma can be clinically important. Ignoring the profound effect of sleep on restorative functions, particularly in posttraumatic situations, would seem inappropriate in the presence of available technology to study sleep in a clinical setting, as well as the existence of data indicating that acquiring this information can be considerably more than just an academic exercise.

NOCTURNAL PENILE TUMESCENCE AND THE DIFFERENTIAL DIAGNOSIS OF IMPOTENCE

The occurrence of full, rigid erections in males is a well-established concomitant of REM sleep. Although NREM erections also occur, they are rare in the neurologically intact organism (Karacan, Salis, and Williams, 1978). Studies by Karacan and colleagues have determined that normally potent males virtually always have evidence of REM-related erections, while patients with vascular and/or neurological dysfunction known to be associated with clinical complaints of impotence commonly have impaired nocturnal penile tumescence (NPT) studies (Karacan, 1982). Thus REM-related erections do have considerable physiological and clinical significance. It would appear that they directly reflect cortically stimulated physiological erectile capability.

The discovery of these facts about NPT has constituted a major breakthrough in the differential diagnosis of impotence. Previously, there was no technique for directly assessing erectile capability, and this rendered the evaluation of impotence an indirect and speculative process. If overt vascular or neurological disease was not apparent, the impotence was generally felt to be psychogenic. In fact, numerous publications in the area of the differential diagnosis have stated that the majority of cases of impotence are psychogenic, and have undoubtedly overlooked a large group of men with erectile dysfunction of undetermined organic etiology (Karacan, Salis, and Williams, 1978).

The erectile response represents the final common pathway of a complex psychophysiological network. In fact, the delicate balance among these factors can be easily disrupted by nearly any condition that compromises the individual's metabolic status. Similarly, a variety of psychological factors must coalesce in order to achieve the appropriate sexual ambience, and disruptions in any of these aspects can also result in a decrease in sexual potency.

The neurological, vascular, and hormonal components of the erectile response have been known for some time, but disruptions of these physiological systems were felt to be relatively uncommon. Recently, a more sophisticated and careful evaluation of patients complaining of impotence has uncovered a variety of organic pathologies that suggest that organic etiologies of impotence exist to a far greater extent than has been previously appreciated (Spark, White, and Connolly, 1980). This investigation documented low testosterone levels and/or elevated prolactin levels in 35 percent of 105 men with a complaint of impotence. Deutsch and Sherman (1980) described impaired glucose tolerance as well as unrecognized diabetes in a group of individuals with impotence who were otherwise asymptomatic. These studies emphasize the importance of a routine endocrine evaluation in patients complaining of impotence.

The well-known vascular and neural components of the erectile response as well as the organic NPT pattern documented in diabetic males complaining of impotence provide considerable support for careful neural and vascular evaluation (Karacan, Salis, Ware, et al, 1978; Velcek, Sniderman, Vaughan, et al, 1980). Routine screening procedures are now available to assess the integrity of both. Penile blood pressures, penile brachial blood pressure indices, pulse volume studies of the penis, and Doppler waveform analysis are being used for the evaluation of pelvic and penile blood flow (Lane, Appleberg, and Williams, 1982; Kempczinski, 1979). Assessment of the bulbocavernous reflex is the most commonly used tool in the evaluation of the sacral neural components of the erectile apparatus (Blaivas, Zayed, and Labib, 1981).

The standard evaluation in our laboratory consists of a history and physical examination; urological evaluation; psychiatric interview; penile blood pressures and indices and Doppler waveform analysis; testosterone, prolactin, fasting and two-hour postprandial blood sugar determinations; and a two-night NPT study in the Sleep Disorders Center. The bulbocavernous reflex at the present time is assessed clinically in the urological evaluation. The interdisciplinary team involved in the evaluation includes a sleep disorders specialist, a psychiatrist, a urologist, and, when indicated, an endocrinologist.

NPT Evaluation

To assess erections adequately it is necessary to place a small mercury strain gauge around both the base and tip of the penis. This permits evaluation of the situation in which an individual may achieve a partial erection that is manifested by normal tumescence at the base of the penis and considerably less than normal tumescence at the tip. An example of such a case would be an individual with Peyronie's disease in whom a plaque in the corpus cavernosum would block blood flow to the distal end of the penis, but would allow normal tumescence to occur at the base. This technique has been shown to provide a reliable assessment of penile expansion associated with erections during sleep. In a recent study published by Fisher et al (1979) in organically impotent males, NPT studies using a similar technique yielded excellent agreement between the nighttime study and the patients' estimates of their daytime functioning. That is, an individual who achieved 15 mm expansion at the base and 12 mm at the tip estimated that during daytime masturbation or attempted intercourse his erections were approximately the same. On the basis of this finding it can be assumed that the NPT study is a reasonably reliable reflection of the individual's true physiological erectile capability.

Until recently, it has not been generally appreciated that the degree of expansion of the penis necessary to achieve a full erection varies tremendously. That is, in one individual 15 mm expansion at the base and 12 at the tip may be a full erection, and in another individual the same degree of expansion may be only a minimal erection. In addition, there may be some dissociation between the degree of expansion and the rigidity achieved. Ultimately, although there is very good correlation in the normal male between expansion and rigidity, there can be discrepancies. Thus an individual can have expansion that would be sufficient to expect a rigid erection, and the actual rigidity achieved would not be sufficient to effect vaginal penetration. To obtain an estimation of the degree of expansion associated with full erection, as well as rigidity achieved, direct assessment of the erection is necessary. It is essential to have at least one full erection evaluated in order to assess other NPT episodes in terms of their degree of normalcy (relative size) for each subject. If this is not accomplished, erroneous and misleading results will occur commonly, particularly in individuals with organic pathology (Fisher, Schiavi, Edwards, et al, 1979; Wasserman, Pollak, Speilman, et al, 1980).

In our experience, it is rare that the full evaluation of an impotent patient reveals a clear-cut functional or organic picture. It seems that the most common situation is a combination of physiological and functional etiologies. This has also been the experience of other groups (Wasserman et al, 1980). This being the case, questions arise concerning the NPT evaluation. For example, to what extent can psychological factors such as anxiety and/or depression and dream content affect the NPT results, and what actually constitutes a normal NPT study?

Although there is controversy concerning the extent to which psychological factors affect NPT, it seems that they would not completely abolish a normal NPT picture. Although an individual may be highly anxious and/or depressed, and this may to some extent alter his normal NPT functioning, it will not abolish the appearance of normal erections during sleep (Karacan, Salis, and Williams, 1978). The question then becomes: If an individual has some normal erectile responses on a two- or three-night NPT study, but they are not enough to be identified with the normal age-matched population, does this constitute a normal study? A somewhat extreme point of view is put forth by Wasserman et al (1980), who stated that the occurrence of a single normal erection in a three-night NPT study is sufficient to indicate that the individual's physiological erectile mechanisms are completely intact.

The answers to questions concerning the erectile response itself certainly depend on the questions asked. Obviously, an individual who achieves a normal erection during sleep has intact physiological mechanisms. But what is the meaning of a study in which an individual achieves far less than normal tumescence time during a two-night evaluation, but clearly has at least one normal erection or has only one full erection and several partial erections? In our experience, such individuals commonly complain of partial erections or ability to achieve a normal erection only infrequently. Here, clearly, nighttime functioning reflects daytime functioning, and suggests an organic etiology. Therefore the patient's complaint must be considered in reaching conclusions about the evaluation. Much research is needed but it appears certain that NPT studies will continue to be a useful and necessary adjunct in the evaluation of impotence.

SLEEP AND GASTROESOPHAGEAL REFLUX

Certain physiological phenomena are characterized by their relative benignity when they occur during waking hours, but they constitute pathophysiological events when they occur during sleep. A prime example of this would be gastroesophageal reflux (GER). This and its clinical correlate, heartburn, are familiar occasional experiences to nearly everyone. Neither is considered a particularly alarming event even when it occurs as many as several times a week; the salubrious effect of commonly used over-the-counter antacid preparations testifies to this. In fact, recent studies involving the monitoring of 24-hour distal esophageal pH have shown that GER is a common event postprandially and frequently occurs in association with belching (Johnson and DeMeester, 1974). Thus even though the clinical manifestation of heartburn may not occur particularly frequently in certain individuals, GER occurs nearly every day in everyone.

The 24-hour distal esophageal monitoring studies by Johnson and his colleagues have elucidated the pathophysiological mechanisms of reflux esophagitis. They have shown not only that daytime GER is benign, but also that frequent GER during the sleeping interval is associated with the development of more severe forms of reflux esophagitis (Johnson, DeMeester, and Haggitt, 1978). These studies strongly suggest that reflux esophagitis is related to the degree of contact between the acid and the mucosa, that is, the amount of time the acidic contents of the stomach are exposed to the esophageal epithelium. Their initial studies demonstrated that daytime GER is associated with rapid clearance of acid from the distal esophagus, demonstrated by relatively rapid return of the esophageal pH to a value above 4. Sleep-related reflux events, although less frequent, tend to last considerably longer and result in a greater degree of acid-mucosal contact. In a study that related these values to actual histological determinations of esophagitis, it was clearly demonstrated that the more severe forms are associated with more frequent nocturnal (supine) GER (Johnson, De-Meester, and Haggitt, 1978).

Subsequent collaborative efforts between our group and Johnson have focused on a number of questions that were posed by the previously cited 24-hour pH studies. Johnson's earlier work strongly suggested that a major issue in the development of esophagitis was not so much the occurrence of GER, but the occurrence of GER during sleep and the attendant prolongation in acid clearance time. These studies did not include polysomnographic monitoring, however, which would allow definitive documentation of sleep-associated reflux events. Thus our studies were designed specifically to document sleep and acid-clearing phenomena. This was accomplished by infusing acid into the distal esophagus and thus producing a drop in the pH to below 4. The acid clearance time is determined by assessing the interval between the drop in pH to below 4 and its return to a value of 4. Our initial study included a group of healthy controls who were studied for two nights in the sleep laboratory and a group of patients with mild to moderate esophagitis who were studied for a single night in the laboratory. The latter group received only infusions (4 to 6) of 15 ml of acid (0.1 N HCl) while the controls were studied for one night during sleep with similar acid infusions and the second night with the same volume of water similarly infused. This allowed determination of the effect of both volume distention and the acidic properties of the substance on clearance and sleep phenomena.

Our study showed virtually no effect of the infusion of water on sleep variables. An infusion of 15 ml of sterile water did not, in most instances, disrupt the subject's sleep. The infusion of acid, however, did produce a marked increase in arousal responses, including brief awakenings from sleep. Arousal responses were generally associated with more rapid clearance times, and in instances where they were not immediately noted or did not occur at all, more prolonged clearance times were documented. Thus it seemed clear that an arousal response was an important component of the response to a noxious stimulus in the distal esophagus (Orr, Robinson, and Johnson, 1981a). Sleep-related infusions were consistently associated with longer clearance times than those occurring under similar circumstances in the pre-sleep waking state. This was true in both patients and in controls, and there was no statistically significant difference between the groups when all sleep-related infusions were considered.

If the amount of wakefulness associated with a particular clearance interval was considered, differences between patients and controls were revealed. It was found that in those acid clearance intervals that were associated with greater than 50 percent waking, patients showed significantly longer clearance times than controls. This indicated that there was no difference between the groups if there was no substantial arousal response to the acid infusion. If, however, there was an arousal response, the patients had longer clearance times than the controls. This occurred in spite of the fact that the swallowing rate was not significantly different between the groups. We felt that this suggested a subtle esophageal motor disorder in the patient group. Subsequent studies are in progress that make use of a specially designed probe to monitor both intraesophageal pH and distal esophageal pressure in order to assess peristaltic values in response to acid infusion during sleep.

Pulmonary Aspiration

The well-known pulmonary complications associated with GER such as pulmonary aspiration and pulmonary fibrosis appear to be directly related to the occurrence of sleep-related GER. Many of the classic symptoms of pulmonary aspiration such as nocturnal cough and morning hoarseness link it directly to the sleeping interval. In a recent study of patients with documented GER with and without symptoms of pulmonary aspiration, Pellegrini et al (1979) noted that individuals with symptoms of pulmonary aspiration had an increased number of GER episodes greater than five minutes in duration during their sleeping interval. In addition, a high incidence of esophageal motor abnormalities (75 percent) was documented in this patient population. It is of interest, however, that a history of heartburn and endoscopic evidence of esophagitis were not consistently identified in the patients with documented aspiration.

An interesting study by Huxley and co-workers (1978) also highlights the importance of the state of consciousness in the occurrence of pulmonary aspiration. These investigators studied normal controls and patients with varying levels of depressed consciousness and infused 10 ml of radioactively labeled saline into the posterior pharyngeal area in 5-ml increments throughout a period of sleep. The following morning the lung fields were scanned. There was a marked increase in positive scans in those individuals with depressed consciousness. In a study using both scintigraphy and 24-hour intraesophageal pH monitoring, two of five patients prospectively studied who had scintigraphic evidence of pulmonary aspiration also had episodes of prolonged acid clearance during sleep in the 24-hour pH study. The other patients with no evidence of aspiration on scan all had normal pH studies (Chernow, Johnson, Janowitz, et al, 1979). Collectively, these data, although inferential in many ways, strongly suggest that GER and the malignant complications of these events, such as pulmonary aspiration and severe esophagitis with stricture, are linked to the occurrence of sleep-related GER.

AROUSALS FROM SLEEP

It is the implicit and unchallenged assumption of physicians and laypersons alike that a restful night of sleep, uncomplicated by arousals and disruptions, is desirable. As a consequence of this attitude, the immediate response of most clinicians to the complaint of disruptive, fitful, poor sleep is to correct this by eliminating arousals from sleep. Most frequently this is done by the reflex prescription of a hypnotic drug. The preceding discussion concerning the complications of GER and other sleep-related pathophysiological events discussed in this book suggest that this attitude can have disastrous effects.

It is a well-known consequence of episodes of obstructive sleep apnea that they are terminated by a brief arousal response. In many instances this produces numerous mini-arousals and a most abnormal and disjointed sleep pattern. Subjectively, the patient responds with a feeling of extreme lethargy and fatigue upon awakening in the morning. Clearly, the patient's sleep is not particularly restful or restorative. Although inherently this is undesirable, consider the consequences of not awakening from sleep subsequent to episodes of obstructive sleep apnea. Obviously this could be life threatening, particularly in individuals who have been sedated or who have a depressed level of consciousness (traumatic head injury, etc.).

Similarly, persons are not uncommonly encountered who awaken numerous times from sleep with complaints related to GER—heartburn, chest pain, and nocturnal cough. Patients with sleep-related GER may, in fact, complain to the physician simply of disruptive, poor sleep, and again the temptation arises to prescribe a hypnotic drug. If the individual's arousal mechanisms are altered, this could result in prolongation of a normal response to acid in the distal esophagus, the attendant complications such as the development of severe esophagitis, and increased risk of pulmonary aspiration (Orr, 1980). Our work has clearly shown that without arousal from sleep subsequent to infusion of acid into the distal esophagus, clearance of this noxious material essentially does not occur.

Swallowing is a volitional act that requires a level of conscious awareness and is a requisite to efficient acid clearance. Our studies have also documented an impressive differential response to acid in the distal esophagus during sleeping and waking. In individuals who have shown no differential responsiveness to acid versus saline infused into the distal esophagus during waking, clear-cut responses to acid in the distal esophagus during sleep have been documented (Orr, Robinson, and Johnson, 1981b). These data support the contention that esophageal responsiveness is substantially altered during sleep in that the esophagus appears to be able to discriminate noxious stimuli more effectively during a state of depressed consciousness, that is, sleep. This has obvious survival value. If the arousal response mechanisms are altered, however, the individual would certainly be placed at increased risk for the considerable complications of GER that may occur during sleep. Additional documentation of this comes from the previously cited study by Huxley et al (1978) in which individuals with depressed consciousness were shown to have an increased frequency of pulmonary aspiration. In Huxley's study it was noted that the normal controls who complained of poor sleep with numerous arousals had uniformly negative lung scans. Those who reported sleeping well had a higher incidence of positive scans.

The arousal response is clearly a complex neurobehavioral event that transcends the normal boundaries of medical specialties and subspecialties. Abnormalities that are ostensibly related to pulmonary or gastrointestinal functioning may indeed be the manifestation of a defective arousal system. Berthon-Jones and Sullivan (1982) have shown that in healthy humans, hypoxia is a relatively ineffective arousal stimulus, and arousal appears to be much less consistently elicited during REM sleep. The authors clearly showed a suppression in the ventilatory response to hypoxia during sleep. Since a relatively low level of arterial oxygen saturation must be achieved to stimulate a response from sleep (only approximately one-half of the normal subjects responded to decreases in arterial oxygen saturation to 70 percent during sleep), hypoxia may not be a particularly effective arousal stimulus, but it clearly functions as a fail-safe mechanism during sleep.

The importance of carotid bodies in the mediation of the arousal response to both hypoxia and hypoxia subsequent to airway occlusion has been demonstrated (Bowes, Townsend, Kozar, et al, 1981; Bowes, Townsend, Bromley, et al, 1981). Further documentation of the importance of the arousal response as a protective response with substantial survival value comes from a study by Sullivan et al (1978), in which responses to laryngeal stimulation (both chemical, through water, and mechanical, by way of balloon distention) were appreciably suppressed during REM compared to NREM sleep. In addition, the authors noted that the protective cough reflex was never fully manifested unless a prior arousal response was noted. Apneic and bradycardiac responses to these laryngeal stimuli were described preceding arousal responses, and again, these were exacerbated during REM sleep.

An interesting integration of the arousal response as a final common pathway of a variety of physiological entities can be accomplished by reviewing much of the literature concerning near-miss or high-risk infants for sudden infant death syndrome (SIDS). For example, GER has been implicated as a pathophysiological mechanism in certain cases of SIDS (Herbst, Book, and Bray, 1978). Defective arousal responses to both hypoxic and hypercapnic stimulation have been documented in a group of near-miss SIDS infants by McCulloch et al (1982). Subsequent siblings of SIDS victims have also been shown to have fewer arousals from sleep and fewer changes in sleep stage, prompting the authors to postulate a defective arousal mechanism in this group of infants (Harper, Leake, Hoffman, et al, 1981). On the basis of these seemingly unrelated data, postulation of a defective neurobehavioral integrative response, that is, arousal response, can possibly account for these data. A defective arousal response could account for a death secondary to GER through failure to produce an appropriate response to aspirated noxious material, which leads to prolonged apnea, bradycardia, and death. A similar defective arousal response could induce a death if there were no appropriate response to decreasing levels of arterial oxygen secondary to a variety of other respiratory and ventilatory abnormalities such as airway occlusion, central apnea, hypoventilation, and so on.

It would appear that arousal from sleep constitutes a basic and fundamental response that has been largely ignored by investigators as well as by clinicians in respiratory, gastrointestinal, and sleep physiology. Further intensive investigation of this response would provide considerably useful information concerning the management of patients with a variety of sleep disorders as well as a better fundamental understanding of the physiology of sleep.

REFERENCES

Adam K, Oswald I. One gram of L-tryptophan fails to alter the time taken to fall asleep. Neuropharmacology 1979;18:1025–27.

Al-Marashi MSH, Freemon FR. Dietary tryptophan effects on the sleep of normal subjects. Waking Sleeping 1977;1:163–64.

Association of Sleep Disorders Centers. Diagnostic Classification of Sleep and Arousal Disorders. 1st ed. Prepared by the Sleep Disorders Classification Committee, Roffwarg HP, Chairman. Sleep 1979;2:1–137.

Bergamasco B, Bergamini L, Doriguzzi T, Fabiani D. EEG sleep patterns as a prognosis criterion in posttraumatic coma. Electroencephalogr Clin Neurophysiol 1968;24:374–77.

Berthon-Jones M, Sullivan CE. Ventilatory and arousal responses to hypoxia in sleeping humans. Am Rev Respir Dis 1982;125:632–39.

Blaivas JG, Zayed AAH, Labib KB. The bulbocavernosus reflex in urology: a prospective study of 299 patients. J Urol 1981;126:197–99.

Bowes G, Townsend ER, Bromley SM, Kozar LF, Phillipson EA. Role of the carotid body and of afferent vagal stimuli in the arousal response to airway occlusion in sleeping dogs. Am Rev Respir Dis 1981;123:644–47.

Bowes G, Townsend ER, Kozar LF, Bromley SM, Phillipson EA. Effect of carotid body denervation on arousal response to hypoxia in sleeping dogs. J Appl Physiol 1981;51(1):40–45.

Brezinova V. Effect of caffeine on sleep: EEG study in late middle-age people. Br J Clin Pharmacol 1974;1:203–8.

Chartrian GE, White LE, Daly D. Electroencephalographic patterns resembling those of sleep in certain comatose states after injuries to the head. Electroencephalogr Clin Neurophysiol 1963;15:272–80.

Chernow B, Johnson LF, Janowitz WR, Castell DO. Pulmonary aspiration as a consequence of gastroesophageal reflux. A diagnostic approach. Dig Dis Sci 1979;24:839–44.

Coble P, Foster G, Kupfer DJ. Electroencephalographic sleep diagnosis of primary depression. Arch Gen Psychiatry 1976;33:1124–27.

Coburn SC, Zeiger DJ, Guilleminault WC, Dement WC. Effects of a hypnotic (flurazepam 30 mg) on respiration and blood oxygen saturation during nocturnal sleep in ten, elderly, "normal" volunteers: a pilot study. Sleep Res 1982;11:81.

Deutsch S, Sherman L. Previously unrecognized diabetes mellitus in sexually impotent men. JAMA 1980;244:2430–32.

Egerton N, Kay JH. Psychological disturbances associated with open-heart surgery. Am J Psychiatry 1964;110:433–39.

Fisher C, Schiavi RC, Edwards A, Davis DM, Reitman M, Fine J. Evaluation of nocturnal penile tumescence in differential diagnosis of sexual impotence: a quantitative study. Arch Gen Psychiatry 1979;36:431–37.

Freemon FR. A critical review of all-night polygraphic studies of sleep medications. In: Kazan F, Harwood T, Rickels K, Rudzik A, Sorer H, eds. Hypnotics. New York: Spectrum, 1975:41–64.

Gillin JC, Duncan W, Pettigrew KD, Frankel BL, Snyder F. Successful separation of depressed, normal, and insomniac subjects by EEG sleep data. Arch Gen Psychiatry 1979;36:85–90.

Gillin JC, Wyatt RJ, Fram D, Snyder F. The relationship between changes in REM sleep and clinical improvement in depressed patients treated with amitriptyline. Psychopharmacology 1978;59:267–72.

Greenwood MH, Lader MH, Kantameneni BD, Curzon G. The acute effects of oral L-tryptophan in human subjects. Br J Clin Pharmacol 1975;2:165–72.

Guilleminault C, Silvestri R. Aging, drugs and sleep. Neurobiol Aging 1982;3(4):379–86.

Harper RM, Leake B, Hoffman H, et al. Periodicity of sleep states is altered in infants at risk for the sudden infant death syndrome. Science 1981;213:1030–32.

Hartmann E. L-Tryptophan as an hypnotic agent: a review. Waking Sleeping 1977;1:155–61.

Hartmann E, Spinwebber CL. Brief communication sleep induced by L-tryptophan: effect of dosages within the normal dietary intake. J Nerv Ment Dis 1979;167(8):497–99.

Heller SS, Frank KA, Malm JR, et al. Psychiatric complications of open-heart surgery. N Engl J Med 1970;282:1015–20.

Herbst JJ, Book LS, Bray PF. Gastroesophageal reflux in the "near-miss" sudden infant death syndrome. J Pediatr 1978;92:73–75.

Huxley EJ, Viroslav J, Gray WR, Pierce AK. Pharyngeal aspiration in normal adults and patients with depressed consciousness. Am J Med 1978;64:564–68.

Johnson LF, Chernik DA. Sedative-hypnotics and human performance. Report no. 81–91. San Diego: Naval Health Research Center, 1981:1–24.

Johnson LF, DeMeester TR. Twenty-four hour pH monitoring of the distal esophagus, a quantitative measure of gastroesophageal reflux. Am J Gastroenterol 1974;62:325–32.

Johnson LF, DeMeester TR, Haggitt RC. Esophageal epithelial response to gastroesophageal reflux, a quantitative study. Am J Dig Dis 1978;23:498–509.

Jouvet M, Pellin B, Mounier D. Polygraphic study of the different sleep phases during chronic disturbances of consciousness (prolonged comas). Electroencephalogr Clin Neurophysiol 1962;14:138–49.

Kagan F, Harwood T, Rickels K, Rudzik AD, Sorer H. Hypnotics. New York: Spectrum, 1975.

Kales A, Bixler EO, Kales JD. Role of the sleep research and treatment facility: diagnosis, treatment and education. In: Weitzman ED, ed. Advances in sleep research. New York: Spectrum, 1974:391–415.

Karacan I. Evaluation of nocturnal penile tumescence and impotence. In: Guilleminault WC, ed. Sleeping and waking disorders. Menlo Park, Calif.: Addison-Wesley, 1982:343–71.

Karacan I, Salis PJ, Ware JC, et al. Nocturnal penile tumescence and diagnosis in diabetic impotence. Am J Psychiatry 1978;135(2):191–97.

Karacan I, Salis PJ, Williams RL. The role of the sleep laboratory in diagnosis and treatment of impotence. In: Williams RL, Karacan I, eds. Sleep disorders: diagnosis and treatment. New York: John Wiley & Sons, 1978:353–82.

Karacan I, Thornby JI, Anch AM, Booth GH, Williams RL, Salis PJ. Dose-related sleep disturbances induced by coffee and caffeine. Clin Pharmacol Ther 1976;20(6):682–89.

Kavey NB, Altshuler KZ. Sleep in herniorrhaphy patients. Am J Surg 1979;138:682–87.

Kay DC, Blackburn ARB, Buckingham JA, Karacan I. Human pharmacology of sleep. In: Williams RL, Karacan I, eds. Pharmacology of sleep. New York: John Wiley & Sons, 1976:83–209.

Kempczinski RF. Role of the vascular diagnostic laboratory in the evaluation of male impotence. Am J Surg 1979;138:278–82.

Kupfer DJ, Foster FG, Reich L, et al. EEG sleep changes as predictors in depression. Am J Psychiatry 1976;133:622–26.

Kupfer DJ, Spiker DG, Coble PA, Neil JF, Ulrich R, Shaw DH. Sleep and treatment prediction in endogenous depression. Am J Psychiatry 1981;138(4):429–34.

Lane RJ, Appleberg M, Williams W. A comparison of two techniques for the detection of the vasculogenic component of impotence. Surg Gynecol Obstet 1982;155:230–34.

Lenard HG, Pennigstorff H. Alterations in the sleep patterns of infants and young children following acute head injuries. Acta Paediatr Scand 1970;59:564–71.

Lester BK, Rundell OH, Cowden LC, Williams HL. Chronic alcoholism, alcohol and sleep. Adv Exp Med Biol 1973;35:261–79.

Miles LE, Dement WC. Sleep and aging. Sleep 1980;3(2):1–220.

McCulloch K, Brouillette RT, Guzzetta AJ, Hunt CE. Arousal responses in near-miss SIDS and normal infants. J Pediatr 1982;101:911–17.

Orr WC. Arousals from sleep: is a good night's sleep really good? Int J Neurosci 1980;11:143–44.

Orr WC, Altshuler KZ, Stahl ML. Managing sleep complaints. Chicago: Year Book Medical Publishers, 1982.

Orr WC, Robinson MG, Johnson LF. Acid clearing during sleep in the pathogenesis of reflux esophagitis. Dig Dis Sci 1981a;26(5):423–27.

Orr WC, Robinson MG, Johnson LF. Swallowing, peristalsis and acid sensitivity during sleep in normals. Gastroenterology 1981b;80:1242 (abstract).

Orr WC, Stahl ML. Sleep disturbances after open-heart surgery. Am J Cardiol 1977;39:196–201.

Passouant P, Cadilhac J, Delange M, et al. Different electrical stages and cyclic organization of post-traumatic comas; polygraphic recordings of long duration. Electroencephalogr Clin Neurophysiol 1965;18:726.

Pellegrini CA, DeMeester TR, Johnson LF, Skinner DB. Gastroesophageal reflux and pulmonary aspiration: incidence, functional abnormality, and results of surgical therapy. Surgery 1979;86(1):110–19.

Rundell OH, Lester BK, Griffiths WJ, William HL. Alcohol and sleep in young adults. Psychopharmacology 1972;26:201–18.

Scrima L, Broudy M, Nay KN, Cohn MA. Increased severity of obstructive sleep apnea after bedtime alcohol ingestion: diagnostic potential and proposed mechanism of action. Sleep 1982;5(4):318–28.

Spark RF, White RA, Connolly PB. Impotence is not always psychogenic. JAMA 1980;243(8):750–55.

Sullivan CE, Murphy E, Kozar LF, Phillipson EA. Waking and ventilatory responses to laryngeal stimulation in sleeping dogs. J Appl Physiol 1978;45(5):681–89.

Velcek D, Sniderman KW, Vaughan ED, Sos TA, Muecke EC. Penile flow index utilizing a Doppler pulse wave analysis to identify penile vascular insufficiency. J Urol 1980;123:669–73.

Vogel GW. A review of REM sleep deprivation. Arch Gen Psychiatry 1975;32:749–61.

Wasserman MD, Pollak CP, Speilman AJ, Weitzman ED. Theoretical and technical problems in the measurement of nocturnal penile tumescence for the differential diagnosis of impotence. Psychosom Med 1980;42(6):757–85.

Williamson J. Paving the way to safe prescribing for the elderly. Geriatrics 1980;35(9):32–39.

Wurtman RJ, Fernstrom JD. Effects of the diet on brain neurotransmitters. Nutr Rev 1974;71:193–200.

CHAPTER 8

The Psychiatric Perspective of Sleep
Ramon Greenberg

Laboratory evidence has demonstrated the interaction between sleep, and in particular, between dreaming and rapid eye movement (REM) sleep, and psychological function. Numerous theories have been presented over the years concerning the function of dreams. This background is reviewed. Clinical applications discussed include the manifestations of sleep pathology and psychiatric illness, the way sleep pathology may affect or be affected by psychological disturbance, and finally, aspects of treatment that relate to interaction between sleep and psychological state.

People have been fascinated by dreams since antiquity. This chapter focuses mainly on the material related to dreams that has been developed since the discovery of the various states of sleep, specifically REM sleep and its relevance to dreaming (Aserinsky and Kleitman, 1953). It is from this modern work that the evidence for psychophysiological interactions in sleep becomes apparent. Studies of both REM deprivation and its effects on psychological function and the responsiveness of REM sleep to psychological events have helped us better understand the function of dreaming. It is important to bear in mind that there is a two-way interaction between waking experience and events during sleep; sleep is not exclusively a psychological or exclusively a physiologic activity.

Rapid eye movement sleep is characterized by a highly activated state of the brain along with extensive inhibition of peripheral sensory and motor activity. It is also marked by concomitant psychological activity, which we know from personal experience and from awakenings from REM sleep in the sleep laboratory as dreams. It is REM sleep, for the most part, in relation to the psychological aspects of sleep, that is the focus of this chapter.

SITE OF BRAIN ACTIVITY IN REM SLEEP

Studies have suggested that REM sleep is triggered in the pons and in fact, some people have spoken of it as pontine sleep (Jouvet, 1961). Although it seems that certain areas of the pons are necessary for development of REM sleep, it is also clear that the cortex is very active, as a matter of fact, more active than during other stages of sleep and as active as in certain stages of wakefulness (Steriade and Hobson, 1976). There are both anatomically specific and nonspecific forms of cortical activation in this process. An example of specific activation would be the increased firing rates among short neurons or association neurons that are activated primarily during REM sleep (Steriade, 1978). Furthermore, there is evidence (at least in animals) that the hippocampus is activated in an unusual way during REM sleep (Passouant and Cadilhac, 1962). An electroencephalographic (EEG) rhythm known as hippocampal theta is found with depth recording in animals during REM sleep and during emotionally activated behavior in the waking state. It is absent during other stages of sleep or when the animal is awake and quiet.

It is hard to conceive of a mental activity such as dreaming without considering cortical function; therefore it seems unlikely that the pons is the sole generator of REM sleep. The effects of damage to the cortex provide evidence that the area plays an integral role in REM sleep. For example, patients who are decorticate maintain periods of REM sleep, but these episodes are markedly abnormal, with impairment of the rapid eye movements associated with REM sleep (Greenberg, 1966). These eye movements have been shown to be connected with the content of dreams (Roffwarg, Dement, Muzio, et al, 1962) in normal subjects. It has been shown more precisely in mammals that damage to the visual association areas of the cortex leads to a decrease in eye movements (Jeannerod, Mouret, and Jouvet, 1965). Finally, studies of patients with lesions of parietal visual association areas show that damage to one hemisphere that leads to an attention hemianopia eliminates rapid eye movements in the direction of the affected visual field (Greenberg, 1966). The interpretation of this particular study has been that, without conscious awareness of one visual field, there is no visual imagery and hence no eye movements toward that field. We return to the implications of this finding later.

FUNCTIONS OF REM SLEEP

The brain is activated in many areas during REM sleep, and evidence shows that all of these areas are part of the total function of REM sleep. An observation of Luria, the Russian neurophysiologist, is relevant in this regard. Exploring functions of the nervous system, Luria (1978) pointed out that biological functions are seldom confined to a single specific area of the body but center on an activity such as respiration, circulation, or perhaps, dreaming. Accordingly, an entire system, and not just its components, is activated during a particular biological activity.

The central nervous system as a whole participates in REM sleep, but this does not explain what function this state serves. The answer has been sought, in part by studying the effects of REM deprivation. This is analogous to the use of ablation in neurological studies of nervous system function. In human studies, REM deprivation is usually accomplished by monitoring the EEG and waking the subject when REM occurs; specific drugs that suppress REM sleep have sometimes been added to this method. Because drugs superimpose nonspecific other effects, EEG monitoring is the main tool for effecting REM deprivation in humans.

For animals, another method has been developed that takes advantage of the marked motor inhibition and motor relaxation during REM sleep. It is known as the "inverted flower pot method" of REM deprivation. Animals (usually rats or mice) are placed on an inverted flower pot partly immersed in water. Non-REM stages of sleep preserve some muscle tone and posture, but if the animal enters REM sleep, associated loss of muscle tone causes either a fall into the water or nodding, which allows whiskers to hit the water and cause awakening. In either case, the animal can be REM deprived.

Studies of REM deprivation have been done with both animals and humans. Earliest studies were for the most part observational with no clear experimental manipulation or design. The first definite finding was that REM deprivation can lead to a marked increase in pressure for REM sleep, that is, a stronger drive toward production or greater resistance against interference with REM. To continue deprivation, more awakenings become necessary on successive nights of deprivation. During recovery nights after deprivation, more REM periods of longer duration occur (Dement, 1960).

Beyond this observation, the first studies in humans showed some sense of heightened psychological turmoil manifested by increases in irritability, anxiety, or eating, or even a suggestion of paranoid thinking. These findings were interpreted to be consistent with the classic notion that dreams function to discharge certain drives, and suggested that a build-up in drives occurs during REM deprivation. Attempts to replicate these findings showed no uniform effect among subjects. These studies, of course, were carefully controlled by awakening subjects during non-REM sleep so that at least there was a comparable number of awakenings for both groups of subjects.

Further observational studies failed to show a consistent effect of REM deprivation until investigators began to develop more specific and testable hypotheses. Among these hypotheses was the idea that information or memory processing occurs during REM sleep. This was based on the observations that dreams seem to have information carried over from the previous day's activity, and furthermore that the cortex is in a highly activated state.

To study the role of REM sleep in dream function, human subjects were studied with more sophisticated techniques including projective tests. In several studies using the Rorschach, evidence for a failure in emotional processing of experience seemed to result from REM deprivation (Cartwright and Ratzel, 1972; Clemes and Dement, 1967; Greenberg, Pearlman, Fingor, et al, 1970). The Rorschach scores also showed impairment of defensive or ego operations. Another study used what has been called tag material (Greenberg, Pillard, and Pearlman, 1972). Subjects were exposed to emotionally disturbing experiences and the effect of REM deprivation on their handling of these experiences was studied. Under normal circumstances adaptation occurs on a second exposure. The deprivation caused failure to integrate the experiences and subjects showed more evidence of continuing anxiety after REM deprivation than when they had normal amounts of REM sleep before the second viewing.

The results of these studies are consistent with the observation that the dreams of people subjected to emotionally significant experiences reiterate or deal with the experiences. This, of course, is one observation that led to the development of the information-processing hypothesis.

A series of studies conducted in Israel suggests a slightly different role for REM sleep and yet in a broad sense also demonstrates its place in adaptation. The REM-deprived subjects were studied for what the investigators called "divergent or creative thinking" (Lewin and Glaubman, 1975). When subjects were presented with a task that measured creative thinking, those without REM sleep showed marked impairment compared to those who were allowed free access to REM sleep. An interesting contrast is provided by another part of the same study in which the effect of REM deprivation on the ability to learn word lists was measured. Learning of words was not impaired by REM deprivation; as a matter of fact, subjects without REM sleep showed better recall of simple word lists than subjects who had REM sleep. This finding has been consistent in a number of studies, and it is important to know that not all kinds of learning are affected by REM deprivation.

Conclusions from the human studies are that REM deprivation affects the integration of emotionally important material or entirely new material, but does not seem to affect learning such things as word lists and other familiar types of experiences.

Complementing the human studies have been many animal studies designed with much larger numbers of subjects in order to explore the problem of information processing. The inverted flower pot method was frequently used. Control animals were placed on flower pots of larger diameters so that with the loss of muscle tone at the onset of REM sleep, they could go into REM sleep without falling in the water. Other studies used a number of drugs that share the common property of suppressing REM sleep but have different nonspecific pharmacological effects. The drugs were used to control for the possible effects of a constricting environment or of discomfort to the animal on the flower pot.

The results of these animal studies paralleled those with humans. For example, REM deprivation did not affect performance of simple tasks such as one-way avoidance in which the animal was exposed to a danger, and it usually took only one exposure before the animal learned that there was a danger. When animals were given more complicated (one might say, more emotionally potent and difficult) tasks, REM deprivation did affect performance. There has now been a series of studies to this effect (Pearlman,

1981). For example, a two-way shuttle box avoidance task, which is somewhat complicated for rats, is affected by REM sleep deprivation with impairment of learning; complicated mazes, discrimination tasks, latent learning, and others in a series of tasks that are complicated for animals to learn have also been found to be sensitive to REM deprivation.

Another important series of animal study borrows from the observation that REM sleep levels are highest in newborn mammals, and some have looked at the role of REM sleep in development. These are clearly quite difficult to do because of the age of subjects, but they point to the fact that REM deprivation will impair the development of certain important psychological functions that seem to be based on early experience. For example, the study used the fact that newborn animals raised in isolation develop abnormally. An hour or so a day of exposure to other animals is enough to undo this isolation effect. If REM deprivation occurs immediately after each exposure to other animals, however, the animals develop as if they were raised in total isolation (Hicks and Moore, 1979). Thus REM deprivation prevents the animal from integrating a new, in this case a developmentally important, experience.

Further evidence for this is provided by studies in rats, showing that REM-deprived animals have a decreased level of emotionality as measured by their experience in an open field running task. This suggests that a normal level of REM sleep is necessary for the development of appropriate reactions within the animals' instinctual repertoire. The finding is somewhat consistent with Jouvet's (1975) speculation that REM sleep is especially important in development in that it brings into play potential instinctual response patterns. The point here is the importance of the interaction between environmental experiences that trigger the development of certain patterns of behavior and an animal's inborn pattern of behavior.

REM RESPONSIVENESS STUDIES

The preceding studies demonstrate the effect of removal of a function. Another way to study function is to examine the responsiveness of that function to certain tasks. Studies in both animals and humans have shown that REM sleep is not a fixed physiological rhythm but seems to respond to demand, much as heart rate or respiration might respond to increased need for oxygen.

The first such studies done in animals involved rats being trained in a two-way shuttle box avoidance task on which performance is impaired by REM deprivation. While they were learning (that is, while they were improving in performance), the rats showed an increase in REM sleep following training trials (Hennevin and Leconte, 1977). When they had learned the task, levels of REM sleep following training sessions fell to normal. Furthermore, individual animals who failed to learn during training showed a failure of this REM sleep responsiveness.

Since that investigation, other animals have been studied with different kinds of tasks such as maze learning, and a similar increase in levels of REM sleep following training has been found. The studies in rats showed a fairly clear rise in REM sleep within the first couple of hours after training trials. When this finding was applied to REM-deprivation studies, it was noted that very brief periods (two to three hours) of REM deprivation were enough to produce the same effect (Pearlman and Greenberg, 1975) as prolonged REM deprivation. Mice studied for REM responsiveness have also shown an increase in REM sleep following training, but in these animals the increase seems to take place over 24 hours.

The REM mechanism also seems responsive in humans. The task presented to them in studies was a more naturally occurring one or was evaluated in terms of a less specific task than, say, shuttle-box learning. Scoring systems were developed to assess patients' mental state prior to sleep. This was evaluated in terms of the putative need for some kind of emotional restoration. In both a group of patients with traumatic war neurosis and a single patient who was undergoing psychoanalysis (Greenberg and Pearlman, 1975a,b), it was found that when the individual showed great emotional disequilibrium prior to sleep, REM sleep appeared earlier in the night than when the patient showed minimal emotional disequilibrium. Thus there was a correlation between emotional pressure and a sign of pressure for REM sleep, the REM latency. It was also shown that when the patient in analysis had evidence of improvement in the disequilibrium between before-sleep and after-sleep samples, levels of REM sleep were higher than when there was no change or when there was impairment or diminution of the equilibrium from presleep to postsleep.

Another series of studies that bears on REM responsiveness was done in students taking intensive foreign-language courses. A small number of students demonstrated that those who improved in their language skills from the beginning to the end of the course had increases in levels of REM sleep during the course, while those who did not show improvement had no increase in levels of REM sleep from before to during the course (DeKoninck, Prouty, King, et al, 1977).

This brief summary of some of the studies designed to relate REM sleep to a function leads us to consideration of some of the suggested functions of REM sleep in dreams.

HYPOTHESES ON THE FUNCTIONS OF DREAMING

Prior to the discovery of REM sleep, the function of dreaming was based mainly on the study of dream content, the major contributor to this scientific study being, of course, Sigmund Freud (Freud, 1953). Freud's major contribution was the demonstration that dreams have a meaning for the subject. Freud went beyond this to develop two interwoven theories of dreaming.

One contends that dreaming is the guardian of sleep. The other, more specific hypothesis says that dreaming is a time for dealing with and attempting to discharge unconscious impulses. This led to his notion of the dream as an opportunity for drive discharge; the solution to the drive would be wish fulfillment.

Freud's theory was clearly based on his model of mental function, which was heavily based upon ideas of drives and energy, and was a kind of hydraulic model. This approach clearly influenced his understanding of the dream. Because he saw a struggle between conscious censoring processes and unconscious forbidden wishes, he attributed the seeming incomprehensibility of the manifest dream to the efforts of a censor and to the process of disguise. He assumed that the major form of thinking in dreams was what he called primary-process, in contrast to waking secondary-process thinking. Primary-process thinking was seen as the language of the unconscious: primitive and illogical. Secondary-process thinking, on the other hand, developed logically. In his classic book, *The Interpretation of Dreams,* Freud discusses these issues using his own and patients' dreams. One, the so-called dream specimen or Irma dream, was especially notable for its illustration of Freud's theory of wish fulfillment. We have reexamined that dream using an approach based on recent work and have reached different conclusions about the thought processes involved in dreams (Greenberg and Pearlman, 1978). Here the elements of disguise and primary process are no longer so central. Instead, it seems important to know the source, in waking life, of the images in the dream and the meaning of those life situations to the dreamer. The coherence and significance of the dream then become more apparent and the underlying processes no longer seem so primitive or illogical.

It is of interest that initial studies of REM sleep suggested similarities or even confirmation of Freud's ideas. This was most striking when it was found that REM deprivation led to a buildup of pressures from REM sleep, as if there were something stored up that had to be discharged. The studies suggest that whatever the nature of the increasing pressure for REM sleep may be, it is not like the build-up of a basic psychodynamic drive. If anything, REM-deprived animals show less drive or intensity (Hicks and Moore, 1979) and one could interpret the psychological tests in humans as also showing evidence of reduced drive (Zarcone, Zokovsky, Gulevich, et al, 1974).

Clinical Considerations

The foregoing discussion provides a background against which to consider the clinical relevance of sleep in the maintenance of psychological health and in understanding and treating patients. If REM sleep and dreams play a particular role in the maintenance of psychic integrity, then paradoxical sleep (REM), in its demonstrable physiological aspects, must play a similar role in animals and in humans. Dreams, however, seem specific to humans. Because in the normal situation dreams seem so closely tied to REM sleep activity, we must assume that they are another aspect of that system's function. With this in mind, some background about dreams and their content may shed a different perspective on findings from electrographical studies of REM sleep.

Integration Process

Studies in sleep laboratories have provided the opportunity to collect large amounts of dream material. These studies have led to increasing focus on the significance of the manifest content of the dream, and it has been shown that this content can be very closely related to issues with which the dreamer is struggling in waking life. This finding should by now sound familiar because it is what we have been suggesting occurs throughout REM sleep: integration of experience.

While dreams can at times have bizarre qualities they also can be quite prosaic. They are a window on the process of integration, a window that at times shows a process working smoothly, with new experiences being organized, confronted, and handled. For example, patients prior to undergoing surgery will show in their dreams evidence of dealing with their concerns about the procedure (Breger, Hunter, and Lane, 1971). A psychoanalytic patient whose dreams were collected in the sleep laboratory showed a very clear connection between the manifest content of his dream and the kind of issues he was struggling with in his analysis (Greenberg and Pearlman, 1975a).

We can go further in deriving information from dreams. One source is the repetitive dream, in particular the repetitive frightening dream, the nightmare. Here one can see not just what the subject is struggling with, but evidence that the person has not been successful in integrating a difficult problem. Instead, it is played over and over again as if it were undigested. This view suggests that dreams show us important dynamic and emotional issues by reflecting what the dreamer is struggling with and how well he or she is succeeding. This is different from the classic analytical idea of drive discharge during dreams, but seems more consistent with the findings from REM sleep studies. The reader should not be misled by these comments into thinking that dreams are therefore easily understood from the manifest content. We must remember that dream language is usually perceptual, mainly pictorial, and not verbal, so that ideas are presented in a language different from our waking language. To comprehend dreams it is necessary to understand the dreamers, their private language, and what defense mechanisms are being used in the struggle to integrate emotionally important issues (Greenberg and Pearlman, 1980). In the nightmare the trauma is clear and the absence of coping is obvious. When a dream accomplishes the task of integration or institution of defenses, the meaning of the dream may be much less obvious. Dream interpretation usually requires collaboration between the dreamer and a perceptive, neutral other person. Because it is so personal, no formulas seem to be useful.

Causes of Sleep Disturbances

Patients who may have sleep troubles seek aid from a physician. Difficulty with sleep may be the stated complaint or there may be other problems. which, as we come to understand them, stem from troubles with sleep. Patients' sleep can be affected by either internal processes or external events. Thus anxiety, pain, or depression that may come from other causes may impair the patient's ability to sleep, and this can create a vicious circle leading to some very manifest and important psychological changes.

We must also be aware that a patient's sleep can be affected by events for which we as physicians are responsible, such as treatment programs, the way we set up hospitals, the way we wake patients, noises from machinery in an intensive care unit, or the drugs we give. All of these factors are going to affect the psychological state of our patients, both directly and through their effects on sleep. It is important that we keep these facts in mind so as to arrive at some guidelines for the clinical applications of our understanding of REM sleep.

Need for REM Sleep

An exception to the generalization that good sleep is probably better for our patients than poor sleep is evidence that REM deprivation for depressed patients can be therapeutic (Vogel, Thurmond, Gibbons, et al, 1975). This notion is upheld by the fact that antidepressant medications also suppress REM sleep. Thus REM sleep or dreams may sometimes work in a maladaptive way in depressed patients: rather than enabling them to integrate new material in a helpful way, the mechanism of REM sleep works to maintain or reestablish an old status quo that is no longer possible. For example, a depressed patient might attempt to deal with a loss by dreaming that the loss does not exist. Such an attempt flies in the face of reality, so that upon awakening the patient is disappointed that the efforts during dreaming have failed. Thus the depressive position is sustained.

Effects of Drug Therapies on Sleep

The positive effect of sleep deprivation in some depressed patients is an exceptional situation, and generally we can assume that if things happen to the patient that impair sleep, particularly REM sleep, there will be a negative impact. From this point of view, we must consider the effects of a number of drugs on sleep, especially those that suppress REM sleep. Until the advent of the benzodiazepines, most sleep medications fell into this group of REM-depressants. (In fact, it seems that many of the drugs used to induce sleep were also addictive, and from physician-prescribed barbiturates and analgesics to patient-prescribed alcohol, we find the connection that all are REM depressants. The physician must be aware of this fact when prescribing such drugs over a long period of time.) When such drugs are discontinued there is often a marked REM rebound, accounting for the marked upsurge in psychological discomfort and frequent appearance of nightmares.

Pertinent to this effect of withdrawal of REM-suppressing drugs is the observation that delirium tremens has been shown to be a manifestation, at least in part, of marked REM deprivation, with the appearance of very high levels of REM sleep prior to the eruption of delirium tremens (Greenberg and Pearlman, 1967). Treatment is directed at helping the patient sleep by using something that no longer depresses REM sleep in order to allow the deficit and prevent the disorder. As mentioned, benzodiazepines add a new dimension to treatment possibilities in that, when given over short periods of time, they allow sleep with a reasonable amount of REM activity. Thus chlordiazepoxide (Librium) has become a very effective treatment for alcohol withdrawal, and can prevent delirium tremens completely if given in adequate doses immediately following cessation of alcohol intake.

The fact that benzodiazepines do not suppress REM sleep makes these the most reasonable drugs to use for control of anxiety or for patients who are having sleep difficulty because of anxiety. One should be aware, however, that over long periods there may be some suppression of REM sleep with these drugs. Also, the benzodiazepines suppress other phases of sleep and therefore should not be used for too long a time or indiscriminately. Furthermore, some of this group of drugs have a rather slow elimination from the body and therefore can build up and lead to drug hangover, sleepiness, or impairment of psychomotor function in the morning. Therefore the clinician should use the shorter-acting benzodiazepines such as oxazepam rather than the longer-acting ones such as chlordiazepoxide or diazepam. Finally, the clinician should be aware that not all sleep difficulty is caused by anxiety, and that for other conditions such as psychotic depression or schizophrenia where sleep disturbance may be very prominent, more appropriate drugs are available to deal with the underlying disorder, and therefore with the sleep difficulty.

Sleep and Psychiatric Disturbance

An enormous amount of research has been done in the search for specific sleep patterns in psychiatric disorders. Depression has been most extensively studied, and while some depressed patients show a shortened REM latency (sleep onset to first REM period), this is true of only a portion of them. Currently, no sleep pattern has been found to correlate with any psychiatric diagnosis, although many patients with psychiatric conditions have trouble sleeping. Thus the sleep disorder generally improves when the underlying condition is treated, but treating the sleep disorder does not treat the primary disturbance. The clinician must not only be aware of the gross effects psychiatric disorders such as depression can have on sleep, but should keep in mind evidence that suggests that dreams themselves may give a clue to the patient's problems. As indicated before, this is most striking for the patient who complains of nightmares.

Nightmares are defined as frightening dreams with content. They are to be distinguished from night terrors, which are sudden terrifying disruptions of sleep without any significant mental content. If mental content occurs in night terrors, it is only a single frightening image. These two conditions differ in terms of their manifestations and have a different physiological substrate. The night terror usually happens early in the night; it occurs as an awakening from stage IV (slow wave) sleep; the nightmare can arise any time during the night but usually occurs later and during awakening from REM sleep.

The night terror has been seen by many investigators as a physiological reaction. Under normal circumstances, arousal from stage IV sleep may lead to a certain amount of temporary mental confusion. The presumption is that somehow the patient with night terrors has even more of this confusion. Clinical experience suggests that people, and certainly adults, who have night terrors usually suffer from significant chronic psychological impairment. It may well be that such vulnerable persons show enormous fear when they awake from stage IV in the normal confusional state. The important point for the clinician is that the appearance of night terrors severe enough to disturb the adult patient probably suggests the need for psychiatric intervention or certainly a psychiatric evaluation. The same thing can be said for other stage IV arousal phenomena such as sleepwalking in adults.

By contrast, nightmares may or may not be of clinical significance. Most people have an occasional nightmare. If we consider what has been mentioned before about dreaming and REM sleep as a time to integrate emotionally important material, the nightmare suggests failure of this integration. The most striking instance of this is the nightmare that is part of war neurosis or poststress syndrome (Greenberg, Pearlman, and Gampel, 1977). In such situations, the sufferer dreams repeatedly of the same event, and the dream is a more or less realistic depiction of the traumatic incident. For some people, nightmares following trauma will gradually change in quality, include other material from the patient's life, and in effect demonstrate that the trauma has been integrated. If the patient has continuous repeated nightmares, however, the chances are that this represents a significant psychiatric problem in that the patient has suffered an emotional injury that has not been handled. Drugs may briefly suppress the manifestations of the trauma but will not be likely to cure it, and again psychiatric intervention is indicated.

Functional Sleep Disorders

Other chapters of this book consider in detail a group of sleep disorders that seem to have a physiological or physical basis and require various kinds of medical intervention, for example, sleep apnea, narcolepsy, and restless legs syndrome. Reports from sleep clinics vary in the incidence of these conditions, but on the whole, when one looks at a large population, they represent a small proportion of the total number of sleep disorders, most of which are functional. This group includes disturbed sleep, as has been described in previous paragraphs, and also excessive sleeping, that is, the desire or need to stay in bed or to sleep for long periods of time.

In either case, one should be aware that most severe sleep disorders are developed from significant emotional problems that require appropriate treatment. The treatment must, of course, be preceded by a careful assessment carried out by a clinician experienced in understanding both sleep disorders and the underlying problems. Sometimes investigation in the sleep laboratory is warranted; in other cases there is more need for the broader clinical perspective that an experienced psychiatrist or psychologist might provide. Most of the functional sleep disorders can be best understood in a clinical interview and will not require any detailed study. A small number, however, can be elucidated in the sleep laboratory, and therefore one should consider obtaining an all-night polygraph recording so as to understand them better. Only after careful assessment can one approach a patient with some assurance that the sleep difficulty will pass, providing some mild sleep medication to help the patient get over a stressful time, or else with the suggestion that the difficulty represents a condition best addressed by psychiatric or psychological intervention. In the last case, the disorder may well be part of a vicious circle in which an underlying process leads to sleep difficulty that causes further failure to cope with life problems and therefore further emotional disturbance. Whether one intervenes by treating the part of the cycle caused by the sleep difficulty or the part caused by underlying emotional difficulties requires individual assessment.

REFERENCES

Aserinsky E, Kleitman N. Regularly occurring periods of eye motility and concommitant phenomena during sleep. Science 1953;118:118–273.

Breger L, Hunter I, Lane R. The effect of stress on dreams. Psych Issues. Vol. 7. New York: International Universities Press, 1971.

Cartwright RO, Ratzel RW. Effects of dream loss on waking behaviors. Arch Gen Psychiatry 1972;27:277–80.

Clemes SR, Dement WC. Effect of REM sleep deprivation on psychological functioning. J Nerv Ment Dis 1967;144:485–91.

DeKoninck J, Prouty G, King W, Poitras L. Intensive language learning and REM sleep: further results. Sleep Res 1977;7:146.

Dement WC. The effect of dream deprivation. Science 1960;131:1705–7.

Freud S. The interpretation of dreams. In: Strachey J, ed. and trans. Standard edition of the complete psychological works of Sigmund Freud. London: Hogarth Press, 1953.

Greenberg R. Cerebral cortex lesions: the dream process and sleep spindles. Cortex 1966;2:357–66.

Greenberg R, Pearlman C. Delirium tremens and dreaming. Am J Psychiatry 1967;124:37–46.

Greenberg R, Pearlman C. A psychoanalytic dream continuum: the source and function of dreams. Int Rev Psychoanal 1975a;2:441–48.

Greenberg R, Pearlman C. REM sleep and the analytic process: a psychophysiologic bridge. Psychoanal Q 1975b;44:392–402.

Greenberg R, Pearlman C. If Freud only knew: a reconsideration of psychoanalytic dream theory. Int Rev of Psychoanal 1978;5:71–75.

Greenberg R, Pearlman C. The private language of the dream. In: Natterson J, ed. The dream in clinical practice. New York: Jason Aronson, 1980.

Greenberg R, Pearlman C, Fingor R, Kantrowitz J, Kawliche S. The effects of dream deprivation: implications for a theory of the psychological function of dreaming. Br J Med Psychol 1970;43:1–11.

Greenberg R, Pearlman CA, Gampel D. War neuroses and the adaptive functioning of REM sleep. Br J Med Psychol 1972;45:27–33.

Greenberg R, Pillard R, Pearlman C. The effect of REM deprivation on adaptation to stress. Psychosom Med 1972;34:257–62.

Hennevin E, Leconte P. Etude des relations entre le sommeil paradoxal et le proces d'acquisition. Physiol Behav 1977;18:307–19.

Hicks RA, Moore JD. REM sleep deprivation diminishes fear in rats. Physiol Behav 1979;22:689–92.

Jeannerod M, Mouret T, Jouvet M. Etude de la motricité oculaire au cours de la phase paradoxale du sommeil chez le chat. Electroencephalogr Clin Neurophysiol 1965;18:554–66.

Jouvet M. Telencephalic and rhombencephalic sleep in the cat. In: Wolstenholme GEW, O'Connor M, eds. The nature of sleep. Boston: Little, Brown & Co., 1961.

Jouvet M. The function of dreaming: a neurophysiologist's point of view. In: Gazzaniga MS, Blakemore C, eds. Handbook of psychobiology. New York: Academic Press, 1975.

Lewin I, Glaubman H. The effect of REM deprivation: is it detrimental, beneficial or neutral. Psychophysiology 1975;12:349–53.

Luria A. Higher cortical functions. New York: Raven Press, 1978.

Passouant P, Cadilhac J. Les rythmes theta hippocampiques au cours du sommeil. In: Passouant P, ed. Physiologie de l'hippocampe. Paris: CNRS, 1962.

Pearlman C. Rat models of the adaptive function of REM sleep. In: Fishbein W, ed. Sleep, dreams and memory. New York: Spectrum, 1981.

Pearlman C, Greenberg R. Posttrial REM sleep: a critical period for consolidation of shuttlebox avoidance. Anim Learn Behav 1975;1:49–51.

Roffwarg H, Dement WC, Muzio T, Fisher C. Dream imagery: relationship to rapid eye movements in sleep. Arch Gen Psychiatry 1962;7:235–38.

Steriade M. Cortical long-axoned cells and putative interneurons during the sleep-walking cycle. Behav Brain Sci 1978;3:465–514.

Steriade M, Hobson JA. Neuronal activity during the sleepwalking cycle. In: Kerkut GA, Phillis JW, eds. Progress in neurobiology. Oxford and New York: Pergamon Press, 1976:155–376.

Vogel GW, Thurmond A, Gibbons P, Sloan K, Boyd M, Walker M. REM sleep reduction effects on depression syndromes. Arch Gen Psychiatry 1975;32:765–77.

Zarcone V, Zokovsky E, Gulevich G, Dement WC, Hoddes E. Rorschach responses subsequent to REM deprivation in schizophrenic and non-schizophrenic patients. J Clin Psychol 1974;30:248–50.

PART III

Polysomnography

CHAPTER 9

Laboratory Assessment of Sleep and Related Functions
George F. Howard III

Polysomnography is a general term that refers to the simultaneous recording of several different physiological variables during sleep. At present, techniques are available for the continuous monitoring of over a dozen such parameters:

Electroencephalogram

Electro-oculogram

Electromyogram

Electrocardiogram

Air exchange (nasal and oral)

Ventilatory movements of the chest and abdomen

Other body movements (by EMG or actigraphy)

Laryngeal sounds

Blood gases (O_2 saturation, CO_2 concentration)

Hormone levels (e.g., cortisol, growth hormone)

Body temperature

Blood pressure

Penile tumescence

Esophageal pH

The clinical utility and indications for studying any of these during a night's sleep are still being investigated and clarified. Nonetheless, sleep laboratories have already made the transition from research to clinical medicine. Polysomnography has clearly proved its value in the diagnosis of several disorders, and we may expect increased use of the technique as physicians outside investigational centers come to recognize its effectiveness.

MEETING PATIENTS' NEEDS

In general, a sleep laboratory must be flexible and capable of adapting its recording scheme to suit the needs of a particular patient. Ideally, all persons undergoing polysomnography should have the benefit of a detailed office evaluation by a clinician associated with the sleep laboratory prior to the study. A differential diagnosis can be formulated and the optimal recording scheme chosen at that time.

Many laboratories offering polysomnography may not be able to interview and examine each patient referred for study. It is imperative, nonetheless, that each patient's clinical data be reviewed prior to the procedure. Selection of an appropriate recording montage* can only be made with knowledge of the patient's symptoms. For example, an individual referred with the complaint of excessive nocturnal awakenings may be monitored differently depending on whether the clinical history suggests central sleep apnea, nocturnal myoclonus, or esophogeal reflux. The referring physician should take primary responsibility for making the clinical concerns known to the personnel of the sleep laboratory and recognize that nocturnal polysomnography is not a single test but a study that is varied and tailored to answer specific questions. When the clinical problem is not clearly delineated by the written requisition, a telephone discussion with the referring physician may be invaluable in deciding exactly how to proceed. Alternatively, a well-trained technologist with a thorough knowledge of sleep disorders may be called upon to interview the patient and modify the protocol according to the patient's complaints. At times, it may become apparent only after the first night's study that modifications in the recording scheme need to be made for succeeding nights so as to understand a particular patient's sleep disorder.

SCHEDULING

Patients generally need to be scheduled for at least two nights in the sleep laboratory, but again, this must be varied from case to case. The patient complaining of headache and confusion on morning awakening may not need to be studied twice if on the first night a nocturnal seizure is recorded. In contrast, an evaluation designed to quantify the degree of disorder in a patient's sleep must be carried out over the course of three or more successive nights to allow the patient to become acclimated to the sleep laboratory. Most people are aware of the fact that they do not sleep as well in a strange bed as they do in their own, even if the strange bed is perfectly

---

*Montage is the word used in electroencephalography to describe a particular recording scheme, the location of the recording electrodes and their manner of connection. Here, the use of montage is expanded to include a description of all variables displayed on the polysomnographic record.

comfortable and in a pleasant setting. This "normal" difficulty is compounded in the polysomnography laboratory. No matter how skillfully attached, the array of monitoring devices and wires routinely employed is bound to cause minor discomfort and irritation. Furthermore, some persons are genuinely apprehensive about the idea of being electronically monitored while they sleep. These factors may serve to alter sleep patterns during the first few nights patients spend in the polysomnography laboratory.

This so-called first-night effect has been investigated by several authors (Schmidt and Kaelbling, 1971; Mendels, Hawkins, 1967; Agnew, Wilse, and Williams, 1966; Rechtschaffen and Verdone, 1964). Most have found that on the first night, sleep is shorter and is interrupted by more arousals than on succeeding nights. The latency to rapid eye movement (REM) sleep is prolonged, and total REM time is abbreviated. In males, the number and rigidity of erections are reduced (Jovanovic, 1969). Consequently, when these measurements are of clinical importance, a single night's study will not suffice.

Off-Site Recording

One possible means of circumventing the problem of first-night effect is to monitor a subject's sleep in his own home. This may be accomplished either by means of a tape recording device or by telephonic transmission of data back to the laboratory. Although elaborate polysomnographical studies cannot be carried out in this manner, simple sleep staging can be reliably done (Rosekind, Coates, and Thorensen, 1978).

Tape recording (Wilkinson and Mullaney, 1976) employs a specially designed, commercially available four-channel cassette recorder. In the laboratory, miniature preamplifiers are affixed to the scalp near the sites of electrode placement and their output is fed directly into a portable cassette recorder. The subject may wear the recorder home on a belt or attached to a shoulder sling. Prior to retiring for the night, the subject places the recorder at the bedside. Later, the tape can be played back onto a video screen in the laboratory at 20 or 60 times real speed. When necessary, samples of the electroencephalogram (EEG) may be frozen on the screen or printed out through a standard polygraph. Electro-oculogram (EOG) and electromyogram (EMG) data are collected simultaneously in a similar fashion to allow for sleep staging.

For the telephonic transmission of sleep data (Riley and Peterson, 1981) a commercially available eight-channel encoder is brought to the patient's home. Preparation of the patient proceeds as it would in the laboratory except that the leads from the recording electrodes are fed directly into the encoder. This device transmits a signal back to the laboratory over a standard telephone connection. A decoding device in the laboratory receives this signal and presents it to the amplifiers of a standard polygraph for immediate printing.

Rosekind and colleagues (1978) have demonstrated that either of these methods may be used to eliminate the usual first-night effect. Thus these techniques may be particularly valuable in documenting a subject's complaint of insomnia and examining the effects of medications on sleep.

BASIC PRINCIPLES AND EQUIPMENT

We have stressed the need for communication between the personnel in a sleep laboratory and the referring physicians, as well as the necessity for changing the polysomnographic protocol depending on the clinical problem being investigated. With this need for flexibility always in mind, one can still outline certain principles that are applicable to all polysomnographic studies.

Responsibilities of the Technologist

The single most important factor in obtaining reliable polysomnographic data is the technologist who performs the test. For this job, a person of considerable skill and endurance is required. First, he or she must be able to deal with patients in a dignified and reassuring fashion. In the presence of a formidable and possibly frightening array of wires and electronic equipment, the technologist must know how to put a subject at ease. This is not only a matter of courtesy. It is important from a practical standpoint since the first-night effect may be minimized by relaxing a subject prior to sleep. Those who perform studies of penile tumescence must be especially capable of maintaining a friendly but strictly professional demeanor. Despite the openness with which sexual issues are discussed in present-day society, men are often still extremely apprehensive about having their erectile function monitored. For reliable data to be obtained, a highly professional rapport must exist between the technologist and the subject.

The job of a polysomnographic technologist is physically and mentally demanding. Often working alone, this individual must be able to remain vigilant throughout the night, make pertinent behavioral observations about the patient, and monitor the performance of all equipment in use. It is necessary to be familiar with common recording artifacts and with signs of instrument malfunction. Furthermore, the technologist must be capable of recognizing and responding to emergency situations. Although back-up medical assistance may be available in a hospital-based sleep laboratory, the technologist must know when to call for aid, for example, in cases of dangerous nocturnal arrhythmias. In cases of seizures or somnambulism, the technologist, being present from the onset, must take responsibility for protecting the patient from injury before help arrives.

Most often suitable polysomnographic technologists come from the ranks of EEG technologists. Those who have been certified by the American

Board of Registration in EEG Technology have already demonstrated the ability to perform EEG studies reliably and to work effectively with patients. To become polysomnographic technologists, however, they must expand their knowledge and skills in a new direction, mastering several other types of monitoring devices and becoming familiar with rather different clinical disorders. Since at this time very few training programs exist for polysomnographic technologists, most of their specialized knowledge must come through private study and work with physicians in charge of sleep laboratories. Some of the major sleep disorder centers in this country periodically offer courses for polysomnographic technologists. These meetings represent a good opportunity for technologists to ensure that their knowledge and skills are on a par with their colleagues in the field. Since 1979 the Board of Registered Polysomnographic Technologists has been examining and certifying technologists who meet its standards. At this time the number of registered technologists is insufficient to fill most of the positions available throughout the country, but it may be anticipated that more will become available in future years.

Polygraph Machines

Numerous options are available in choosing a recording device for clinical sleep studies. A large polygraph equipped with 12 alternating current (AC)- and one or more direct current (DC)-coupled amplifiers will allow great flexibility in recording, but smaller polygraphs or standard EEG machines may be adequate for many studies. The chief drawback of the standard EEG machine is its inability to record constant or very slowly varying signals. The reason for this can be understood by examining some of the basic principles involved in recording bioelectrical potentials.

Each channel on a polygraph machine employs a multistage amplifier that senses the difference in electrical potential between its two inputs and responds by producing a proportional but much larger electrical signal at its output terminals. This larger signal is generally used to drive a mechanical ink writer. The tracing that results is a graphic display of the difference in electrical potential between the amplifier inputs versus time.

The manner in which the input signals are connected to the first stage of the amplifier is crucial (Figure 9.1). In DC-coupled systems, no capacitor is placed in the input circuit. Consequently, any difference in electrical potential between the inputs, even a nonvarying one, will reach the amplifier. In AC-coupled systems, the input circuit contains a capacitor. When an electrical potential is applied across the amplifier inputs, the capacitor begins to fill with electrical charge and tends to create an electrical potential opposite to the one applied. If the applied electrical potential remains constant after it has been turned on, eventually the capacitor will arrive at a steady state in which it possesses enough charge to balance exactly the applied

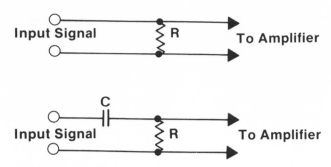

Figure 9.1. Schematic drawings to illustrate DC coupling and AC coupling.

potential difference. At that point, no further current will flow in the amplifier input circuit. The polygraph will read zero even though a steady input potential difference is still present.

For input potentials that vary only slowly, the effect of the capacitor is to attenuate the amplitude of the signal entering the amplifier. On the other hand, for extremely rapidly varying electrical signals, the capacitor has no apparent effect. This is because the charge on the capacitor and the resulting potential difference across it do not build up or decline instantaneously but in an exponential fashion. The rate of build-up (or decline) depends on the size of the capacitor, C, and the resistance, R, to current flow in the input circuit. The details are such that the product of C and R has the units of time. This value, called the time constant, characterizes the speed with which changes occur in a specific input circuit. In particular, R times C is the time it takes the capacitor to build up from zero to 63 percent (or fall from 100 to 37 percent) of its maximal charge when a given voltage is applied.* When the input potential varies rapidly compared to the time constant, the capacitor never has enough time to build up or lose much charge, and no opposing potential difference develops in the input circuit. As a result, the amplifier sees no attenuation of the applied potential.

The practical consequence of these considerations is that either AC- or DC-coupled amplifiers can be used to measure varying electrical signals, but only the latter can be used for constant or slowly varying signals. In general, as the time constant of the AC-coupled amplifier is increased, the attenuation of low-frequency signals decreases and the amplifier behaves more and more like a DC-coupled system.

---

*These figures are obtained by solving the differential equations which govern such circuits. The exact numbers are:

$$1 - e^{-1} \approx 63 \% \text{ and } e^{-1} \approx 37\%$$

where e is the base of the natural logarithm function.

The problem of recording eye movements can be used to illustrate these ideas. Because of a difference in electrical potential between the retina and the cornea, an electrical field always exists around the eye (Figure 9.2). When the eye is in motion, electrodes about the orbit experience a changing electrical field. The resulting difference in electrical potential between a pair of electrodes varies in time and can be recorded through either an AC- or a DC-coupled amplifier. When the eye is at rest, the electrodes experience a constant difference in electrical potential, the magnitude of which depends on the position of the globe. A DC-coupled system is able to record such static differences, but an AC-coupled amplifier yields an output of zero for any eye position that does not vary. Thus eye position can be recorded only by DC-coupled amplifiers, but eye movement can be monitored through either system. In sleep studies where only eye movements are important, the EOG can be adequately recorded by an AC-cou-

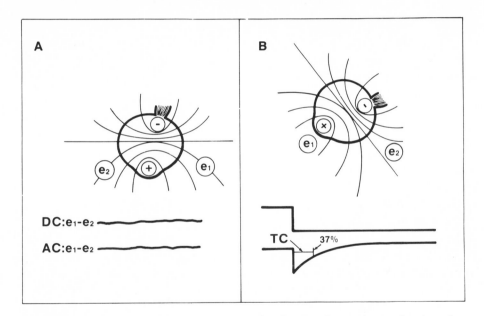

Figure 9.2. (A) A cross section of a globe is seen from above showing the electrical potential difference between retina and cornea. Some isopotential lines (lines that connect points of equal electrical potential) have been drawn in. Two recording electrodes, e_1 and e_2, are placed on either side of the globe anteriorly. Both the AC- and DC-coupled polygraphs record zero because the electrodes have been placed on the same isopotential line. (B) The eye has instantaneously turned toward electrode e_1. Now the two electrodes are not on an isopotential line, so the DC-coupled polygraph displays a non-zero signal, which is proportional to the angle of the new eye position. The AC-coupled system responds initially in a like manner, but since the eye position then remains constant, the AC-coupled signal declines as charge builds up on the capacitor within its input circuit.

pled amplifier. The same is true for most other variables of importance in clinical sleep studies. Exceptions to this rule include oxygen saturation, penile tumescence, body temperature, and esophageal pH. In studies requiring a graphic display of these values, a DC system must be employed. The EEG, EMG, and other determinations such as air flow and ventilatory movements vary sufficiently rapidly to be recorded through AC-coupled equipment. This simplifies the recording of polysomnographic studies because DC-coupled systems are intrinsically less stable. In addition, electrodes acceptable for DC recording require special care. These issues are discussed further in a later section.

An advantageous feature present on polygraph machines but absent on many EEG machines is a choice of slower paper speeds. The standard recommendation is to use a paper speed of 15 mm per second when sleep is to be staged (Rechtschaffen and Kales, 1968). For certain studies, slower speeds can be employed without a significant loss of clarity. In such cases, great conservation of paper may be achieved by recording the study at paper speeds of 10 mm or even 6 mm per second.

Polygraph machines with fewer channels require greater care in selecting the variables to be recorded. One set montage cannot be used nightly without the risk of overlooking relevant diagnostic data. The considerations involved in choosing a certain recording scheme are discussed presently. For the discussion of montages to be unambiguous, standard EEG nomenclature is reviewed first.

EEG Nomenclature and Conventions

Scalp electrodes are positioned according to the international 10-20 system in which the scalp is measured in three planes: one longitudinal, one transverse, and one circumferential. Each dimension is divided equally into units of 10 or 20 percent of the whole, as shown in Figure 9.3. Lines are imagined to connect these points of division both transversely and longitudinally. The intersections of these lines are given standard names, as shown. Note that all odd numbers refer to the left side of the scalp and all even numbers to the right. In addition to the scalp positions, the earlobes are labeled as A_1 and A_2. For purposes of this discussion, we will also define locations about the eyes: LOC and ROC for positions just lateral to the left and right outer canthi respectively, LOC' for the position 1 cm above LOC, and ROC, for the position 1 cm below ROC (see Figure 9.5 (A) on p. 209).

The inputs of an amplifier are designated I_1 and I_2 and written with a hyphen, e.g., C_3-A_2. By convention, polygraphs are wired so that an upward pen deflection will result when I_1 is more negative than I_2 and vice versa.

Recordings made between two scalp electrodes are frequently referred to as bipolar in distinction to those made between scalp electrodes and a common nonscalp reference such as the ear or neck. The latter were formerly called unipolar under the mistaken notion that only the scalp elec-

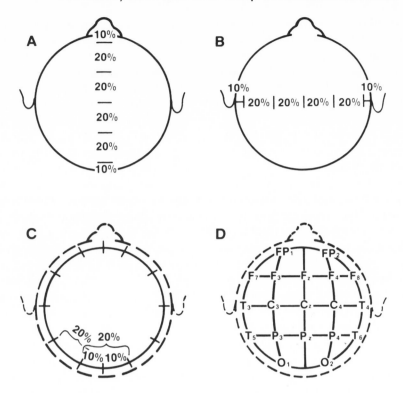

Figure 9.3. The international 10-20 system. A longitudinal measurement is made in *A* from nasion to inion. A transverse measurement is made in *B* from ear canal to ear canal. The circumferential measurement is made in *C* through the 10 percent marks determined in *A* and *B*. The 10 and 20 percent marks are connected and their intersections labeled in *D*.

trodes were recording brain activity and that the nonscalp electrode was electrically inactive. It is now recognized that any of the commonly used reference sites may be influenced by brain activity, and so the old words bipolar and unipolar are no longer appropriate. The terms scalp-to-scalp and scalp-to-common reference or referential should be used instead.

The characteristics of each of these two types of recordings are somewhat different and need to be kept in mind. The most important distinction between them is in common-mode rejection. Any electrical potential that affects both input electrodes at the same time will be cancelled to some extent. This is due to the fact that amplifiers measure the difference in potential between I_1 and I_2. Consequently, an electrical field that has a wide distribution and whose magnitude varies little from point to point on the scalp will be largely cancelled in scalp-to-scalp recordings. Common reference montages will show such a field to better advantage because of a generally greater interelectrode distance and less cancellation. Local electrical potentials such as cortical spike foci are better seen by connecting scalp electrodes one to another in chains. In this way, the local disturbance will affect I_1 to a greater extent in some channels and I_2 in other channels. Phase reversal between channels will be evident over the source of the local potential (Figure 9.4).

Sleep Staging Montage

Sleep staging is achieved by examining EEG, EMG, and EOG data simultaneously. The recommended minimum number of data channels for accurate sleep staging is four (Rechtschaffen and Kales, 1968): one EEG channel (C_3-A_2 or C_4-A_1), one EMG channel (under the chin), and two EOG channels (LOC'-A_2 and ROC,-A_2).

The recommended EEG channel invariably will display sleep spindles and K-complexes in an unambiguous fashion, so the presence of stage II can be readily determined. Usually the posterior alpha activity is seen well enough on this channel to judge the onset of drowsiness as well; however, this derivation may prove inadequate when multiple transitions from stage W (wakefulness) to stage I are present. In such cases the addition of O_1-A_2 will clarify matters. Some authors (Cooper, Osselton, and Shaw, 1980) suggest the scalp-to-scalp derivation Cz-Oz. Both the posterior alpha activity and the central sleep activity will generally be seen well in this one channel. This disadvantage of using this system is that the accepted standards for staging sleep specify the C_3-A_2 (or C_4-A_1) derivation, so studies scored with a scalp-to-scalp montage will not be completely comparable.

The EMG recording is made from a pair of electrodes situated just behind the lower border of the mandible near the midline. An alternative location is adjacent to the hyoid bone. Although here a decrease in muscle tone with REM onset is less consistent, this position had the advantage of being closer to the heart. As a result the ECG can be recorded on the same channel, conserving space when an extra amplifier is not available (Jacobson, Kales, Zweizig, et al, 1965).

The recommendation of a two-channel montage for monitoring eye movements can be understood by examining the behavior of this system in detail. When the eyes move conjugately to the left, LOC' becomes relatively more positive and ROC, more negative. Assuming that the common reference A_2 stays at approximately the same potential, the channel LOC'-A_2 will show a downward deflection and ROC,-A_2 an upward deflection. When recorded on two adjacent polygraph channels, a striking convergent phase reversal results. Conjugate eye movement to the right results in a divergent phase reversal. Vertical eye movements cause similar responses (Figure 9.5).

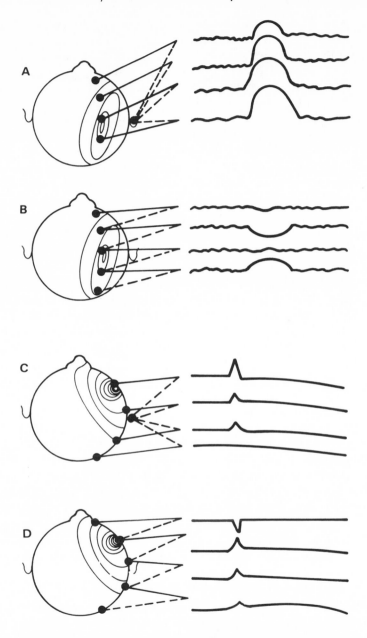

Figure 9.4   Common reference recording of a large slow wave (A). Demonstration of the cancellation that scalp-to-scalp recordings may exhibit when the potential of interest is widely distributed (B). Common reference recording of a sharp wave (C). Demonstration of the clear localization of a sharp wave by phase reversal in a scalp-to-scalp montage (D).

When greater economy of channels is required, the two EOG tracings can be condensed into one. The simplest means of accomplishing this is to refer one of the given eye electrodes to the other. This montage is sensitive to both vertical and horizontal conjugate eye movements, but brain activity often contaminates the recording and complicates interpretation. Here the phenomenon of common-mode rejection can be used to advantage. If the electrodes are placed in the same horizontal plane, that is, at ROC and LOC (Wells, Allen, and Wagman, 1977), greater cancellation of brain activity will generally occur. Diminished sensitivity to vertical eye movement will result, but this is unlikely to detract from the recognition of REM episodes. A more complicated one-channel EOG has been described (Hord, 1975) where four electrodes are used: two above the inner canthi and two below the outer canthi. The lateral electrode from one eye is connected to the medial electrode of the opposite eye and the combination fed into one input of the EOG amplifier. The other pair of electrodes serves as input number two. Considerable common-mode rejection of brain activity will result, but sensitivity to vertical eye movement will not be any greater than with the simpler ROC-LOC montage. Either of these one-channel systems can be employed when no extra channels can be afforded for the EOG, but neither can give the striking phase reversals that make conjugate eye movement so easy to detect on the recommended two-channel, common reference montage.

Preparation of the Patient

The techniques used in recording a reliable EEG during the day apply equally well at night in recording a polysomnogram. The application of electrodes must be even more carefully performed due to the longer period of recording and the greater likelihood of patient movement. The standard 10-20 system positions are used as described. The skin is first cleansed with a commercially available solution. Such products generally contain abrasive particles that remove oil and the outermost layers of skin so as to achieve skin electrode impedances below 5,000 ohms. Overzealous cleansing with abrasive solutions can lead to painful sores, so care is required. Standard electrodes are applied at the chosen EEG, EMG, and EOG locations. As usual in EEG practice, each electrode is filled with a conductive gel and firmly secured by placing a small gauze pad soaked with collodion over the electrode; the adhesive is dried with compressed air. For those with sensitive skin, plastic tape may be used on the face instead of collodion. Some authors recommend electrode paste, which serves as both conduction medium and adhesive, but this technique should probably be reserved for shorter daytime studies and patients who for some reason cannot tolerate collodion. In spite of the best technique, electrodes may come loose during the night due to

A

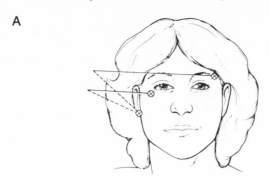

B   **Horizontal eye movements**

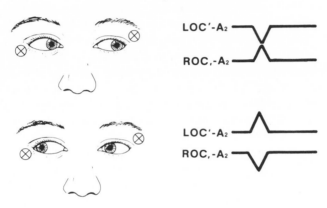

Vertical eye movements

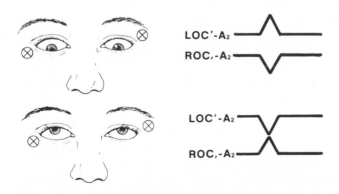

Figure 9.5. (A) Position of the eye electrodes LOC' and ROC,. (B) The response of the system is shown for horizontal and vertical eye movements.

patient movement. It is wise therefore to apply some back-up electrodes at the start of the study. These should include an extra EMG electrode under the chin, the other ear, and the opposite central and occipital scalp electrodes.

Various types of commercially available electrodes will perform adequately since the EEG, EMG, and EOG are all recorded through AC-coupled systems, but it is wise to be aware of the influence electrodes can have on recording fidelity. To understand these effects, the properties of recording electrodes need to be examined.

When two dissimilar electrical conductors (e.g., a metal electrode and an electrolyte gel) are placed in contact, ions diffuse from one medium to the other and create a difference in electrical potential between the electrode and the gel. A double layer of oppositely charged ions forms at the point of contact. If a pair of like electrodes is used in each channel, electrical potentials at the two places where electrode and gel touch will tend to cancel each other. Impurities may lead to inexact cancellation, however, and a net electrical potential may be fed into the amplifier input. This potential may vary slowly over the time of the recording session. Such a slowly varying signal will be effectively blocked by an AC-coupling capacitor, but in DC-coupled systems it will reach the amplifier and result in sway of the electrical baseline.

When an external electrical potential is applied across the interface of an electrode and electrolyte gel, considerable impedance to current flow may result from the electrical double layer. The magnitude of this impedance will depend on the frequency of the applied signal, just as it does for a capacitor. Slowly varying potentials will be severely attenuated, while rapidly varying signals will suffer almost no apparent effect. Electrodes that form such an electrical double layer are called polarizable. They in essence turn DC coupling into AC coupling. Gold, silver, and stainless steel electrodes all act in this way to different degrees depending on their size and shape. The smaller the electrode surface area, the more pronounced its capacitative effect.

Other electrodes such as those of silver coated with silver chloride do not build up an electrical double layer and are therefore called nonpolarizable or reversible. Even small electrodes of this type do not severely attenuate constant or slowly varying potentials. Electrodes of this type are the only ones that may be employed in DC recordings, but because of their smaller size they may be preferred even in AC-coupled montages for recording from the face, for example. The upkeep of silver/silver chloride electrodes is more difficult than, for example, gold, because of the necessity for maintaining a uniform silver chloride deposit on the surface of the electrode. Thus for many applications other than DC recordings, polarizable electrodes are often used.

Whatever electrodes are decided upon, all their wires should be gathered toward the top of the head and tied in one bundle before they leave the patient and the bed. In conditions where excessive movement is expected, such as somnambulism or seizures, it may be wise to wrap the patient's head in gauze to secure the scalp electrodes further. Longer lead wires may need to be used, and there should be no fixed attachments to the bed to restrain either the electrode box or its connecting cable. The room in which the study is to be performed should be insulated from excessive external noise and light. The polygraph should be located in an adjoining room and a small window should connect the two rooms, so that the technologist may observe the patient directly throughout the study. Electrical junction boxes in the wall receive data from the patient and pass it on to the adjoining room. Alternatively, signal cables can be brought out to the polygraph through a porthole in the wall, but the aperture must be soundproof.

Although not absolutely essential, a video monitoring and recording system is highly desirable in many sleep studies. It provides a clearer documentation of the patient's behavior than a few hurriedly scribbled notes by the technologist. For illumination, an infra-red lighting system may be used, or the room light may be turned up slightly after the patient is asleep. To correlate the videotape with the polysomnogram, a special-effects generator is generally required. The polysomnogram can be placed under a video camera and the tracing added to the picture of the patient being simultaneously recorded. With other special-effects systems, a few channels of the polysomnogram can be superimposed directly on the video picture electronically. With either method, the date and time should also be continuously shown on the screen and recorded.

METHODS OF MONITORING

Ventilatory Effort

The first two methods measure intrathoracic pressure or respiratory muscle activity directly. The remainder monitor ventilatory effort by measuring chest and abdominal movement.

Esophageal Pressure Sensors

Esophageal pressure sensors are commercially available in catheter-tip or balloon types. Either device must be guided through the nose (or mouth), swallowed by the patient, and allowed to remain in the distal esophagus during the course of study. The air-filled output tubing is connected to a pressure/voltage transducer and the resulting signal is displayed on a polygraph. A continuous tracing of changes in intrathoracic pressure results. When properly calibrated, a DC amplifier will allow absolute pressure values to be recorded, while an AC system will show only variations of pressure. Instead of a specially designed esophageal balloon, a Swan-Ganz catheter may be used (Gillies, Larkin, Guy, 1981).

Placement of such devices generally requires preparation of the nasal and pharyngeal mucosa by spray application of a local anesthetic. The somewhat invasive nature of the placement procedure and the inability of some patients to tolerate it make this method of monitoring ventilatory effort less than optimal for routine use.

Intercostal Electromyography

The intercostal EMG can be recorded with surface electrodes affixed to the chest wall, but obesity may interfere with the use of this technique.

Pneumatic Devices

These instruments employ a distensible air-filled bladder or cuff very similar to that of the sphygmomanometer. The cuff is held snugly to the anterior chest or abdominal wall by a strap that attaches to either end of the cuff and encircles the patient. When the torso expands, the cuff is distended and pressure within the bladder rises. A tube conveys pressure changes within the air-filled bladder to a pressure/voltage transducer at the bedside. The resulting electrical signal may be displayed on a standard AC or DC polygraph. Unfortunately, data from such devices may be seriously distorted by any change in the position of the cuff or movements by the patient.

Strain Gauges

The electrical resistance through a column of mercury (or other liquid conductor) varies directly with the length and inversely with a cross-sectional area of the column (Shapiro and Cohen, 1965). If mercury is placed in a distensible tube, stretching the tube will increase resistance through the enclosed liquid metal by increasing the column length and decreasing the cross-sectional area. When appropriately electrified and connected to an AC or DC amplifier, such tubes may be strapped to the chest or abdominal wall and used to sense changes in the torso's circumference. While these are relatively inexpensive devices, their performance depends greatly on stable positioning. Even small amounts of patient movement may lead to excessive artifact.

Impedance Pneumography

If a high-frequency electrical signal is applied to the chest wall by means of two surface electrodes, the electrical impedance experienced by that signal as it passes between the electrodes will vary depending on the position of the chest wall. This observation led to the development of impedance pneumography.

Numerous variations in instrumentation have been made, but all such devices are based on the same theoretical foundation (Pacela, 1981). In practice, a high-frequency oscillator is used to produce an AC carrier signal of constant strength. This current is applied directly to the chest wall. The voltage drop across the torso varies with movement and serves to modulate the amplitude of the carrier signal. These modulations of amplitude may be picked up from the body surface by either the input electrodes themselves or a separate pair of recording electrodes. A demodulator then converts the variations of carrier signal amplitude into a form suitable for display on a standard AC polygraphy.

Respiratory physiologists have shown considerable interest in the technique of impedance pneumography because of its potential for yielding quantitative data on changes in lung volume. Reliable quantitative information may not be obtainable if the subject changes position, however, either turning sideways or sitting upright (Ashutosh, Gilbert, Auchincloss, et al, 1974). For most applications of polysomnography, precise measurements of lung volume are not required. Impedance pneumography is an adequate technique for qualitatively monitoring ventilatory effort. The simplicity of commercially available devices and the relative stability of this method are significant advantages. The surface electrodes attached to the chest wall may be used to record the electrocardiogram (ECG) as well as changes of chest impedance. The two signals may be displayed together in the same polygraph channel and thus leave room for recording an additional signal.

Magnetometers

An electrified coil of wire produces a magnetic field, and the strength of that field declines with increasing distance from the coil. Any other coil placed within the magnetic field will develop a current proportional to the strength of the applied field. If the excitatory coil is placed on the posterior wall of the torso and the sensing coil on the anterior wall, the current induced in the second coil may be used to monitor the anteroposterior diameter of the chest or abdominal cavity. An instrument of this type is called a magnetometer. Unfortunately, such devices are highly sensitive to changes in relative position of the coils, and so they are not generally employed in sleep studies. Theoretical and experimental work has demonstrated the possibility of recording quantitative data from such instruments, but as with impedance devices, any change in the patient's position necessitates recalibration (Ashutosh et al, 1974).

Inductive Plethysmography

The most recent advance in ventilatory monitoring is inductive plethysmography. A wire sewn into an elastic band of cotton mesh encircles the patient's chest or abdomen. When the torso expands, the circle of wire enlarges and the electrical inductance of the loop is changed. An alternating current applied to such a device experiences a variable inductive reactance related to movement of the torso. Appropriate electronic circuitry permits a standard AC or DC polygraph to monitor ventilatory effort by this means.

This technique turns out to be much more powerful than those described above; it can supply quantitative data on tidal volume. To understand how, some facts about ventilatory dynamics need to be considered.

An increase in lung volume can be divided theoretically into two independent parts, a thoracic and an abdominal component—one related to expansion of the rib cage and the other due to flattening or depression of the diaphragm (Konno and Mead, 1967). The two components can be measured separately. Rib cage expansion is manifested by increased thoracic dimensions and flattening of the diaphragm by increased abdominal dimensions. Because the height of the torso is fixed, the volume of either the chest or the abdominal components vary directly with cross-sectional area. Circumference and anteroposterior diameter are more readily measured, but neither adequately reflects lung expansion because these values bear an inconstant relationship to the torso's cross-sectional area. This is so because changes in a subject's position distort the shape of his chest and abdomen. (A circle and an oval may have the same surface area, but clearly their circumference and anteroposterior diameter will be different due to their different shapes.)

In contrast to strain gauges and magnetometers, inductive plethysmographs produce a signal directly proportional to the encircled area, not its circumference or diameter (Watson, 1980). Consequently these are the preferred devides for measuring lung expansion since they allow quantitative data on lung volume to be obtained regardless of the patient's position. The instrument is calibrated so that the algebraic sum of the chest and abdominal signals will be equal to the volume of air exchanged through the mouth and nose. If the airway is obstructed, no air will be exchanged, and any change in chest volume will be associated with an opposite change in abdominal volume, that is, the sum of the two will be zero.

To the polysomnographer, this means that complete ventilatory monitoring can be accomplished with only two bands around the torso and three recording channels: one for thoracic movement, one for abdominal movement, and one for the sum. An independent measure of air flow is theoretically unnecessary. The presence of apnea can be ascertained by observing the tracing that sums chest and abdominal movement because this reflects total air exchange. Flattening of all three tracings indicates central apnea. On the other hand, continued but opposite movements of the chest and abdomen at a time when the sum tracing is flat (no air movement) indicate obstruction of the airway. One cautionary word should be given: for inductive plethysmography to be used in this fashion, careful calibration is required, as described by Cohn et al (1978). For certain patients, calibration may be difficult or impossible, and a separate air-flow monitor should be employed.

For all of the preceding types of chest and abdominal movement monitors, summation of the chest and abdominal signals does not necessarily reflect air flow since accurate volume measurements cannot be made by these instruments when the patient is free to move around in bed. All of these other methods must be employed in conjunction with an independent air-flow monitor such as those to be described below.

Air Flow

Thermistors and Thermocouples

Thermistors and thermocouples are the least expensive equipment available to monitor air flow. Thermistors are small glass beads that react to changes in temperature by changing their electrical resistance. When electrified by a standard 1.5-V battery, the voltage drop across a thermistor varies with temperature. Expired air warms the thermistor, producing a signal that can be displayed on an AC- or DC-coupled polygraph. Thermocouples consist of two dissimilar metals in electrical contact. As mentioned earlier in the discussion about electrodes, a potential difference develops at the contact point between unlike conductors. The magnitude of this difference depends on temperature. Thus thermocouples spontaneously produce a low-voltage signal that varies with changes in temperature. No external power source is required for operation.

Both thermistors and thermocouples are small enough and lightweight enough to be placed directly into the flow of a subject's expired air. In polysomnography the measurement of interest is the combined air flow from mouth and nose. This may be measured in various manners. Often, separate thermistors are taped to the face, one projecting into the stream of expired air from the mouth and another under one nostril. Since air flow may differ from one nostril to the other during the course of the night, two nasal thermistors are preferable for complete recording. Alternatively, a hook-shaped holder may be used to direct air flow from both nostrils past a single thermistor. These devices are taped onto the bridge of the nose and cause no particular discomfort. An oral thermistor, as it projects from the side of the mouth into the path of oral air flow, is generally held in place only by the stiffness of its own wire. Movement by the patient may disturb the position of the thermistor. Since these devices are extremely sensitive to minor changes in the angle at which they encounter air flow, loss of signal may result from a change in position.

Thermistor position may be stabilized by attaching the device to a cannula or mask. With a simple oxygen mask a single thermistor can be rigidly situated in the path of combined nasal and oral air flow (Fisher, Garza, Flickinger, et al, 1980). The mask set-up is relatively resistant to patient movement, but if displaced, it can be easily readjusted, often without disturbing the patient.

Carbon Dioxide Detectors

A much more expensive means of monitoring air flow is to measure the carbon dioxide content of air present around the mouth and nose. This method also requires that the patient wear a lightly fitting mask into which a probe is placed. The probe may be connected to a standard carbon dioxide measuring device employing infra-red or mass spectrometry. For clinical polysomnography, no particular advantage is conveyed by this method.

Flow Transducers

Another means of monitoring air flow is to have the patient breathe through a pneumotachygraph. This device samples the air pressure within a tube attached to the patient's face mask and transmits changes in pressure through a thin plastic tube to a pressure/voltage transducer at the bedside. The pressure inside the tube varies with each inspiration or expiration, producing a signal that can be displayed on a standard AC polygraph.

Laryngeal Sound Recorders

A newly described method of monitoring air flow employs sound recordings from outside the larynx. A stethoscope head is affixed to the lateral surface of the neck and its output is air-coupled to a conventional microphone without any preamplification. After appropriate filtering, rectification, integration, and amplification, a display of laryngeal sound intensity is obtained that can be used to document periods of apnea. The authors of this technique (Krumpe and Cummiskey, 1980) have pointed out that several disadvantages of the other air-flow monitoring methods are avoided. The problem of maintaining precise detector position and the discomfort of a mask are eliminated.

Oxygen Saturation

To evaluate the severity of apneic episodes, the degree of oxygen desaturation must be recorded. While it is possible to place an indwelling arterial catheter and take serial blood samples throughout the night, the noninvasive technique of transcutaneous oximetry is greatly preferred. Commercially available instruments shine red light through the external ear (Figure 9.6) or a finger. For certain wavelengths, the ability of hemoglobin to transmit

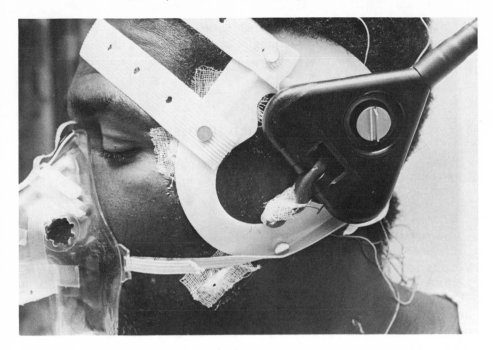

Figure 9.6.   An ear oximeter strapped into place.

light depends upon the molecule's oxidation-reduction state. By comparing the percentage of light transmitted for different wavelengths, a value for hemoglobin oxygen saturation can be calculated as a percentage. The oximeter console should be situated so that the readout will be visible to the polysomnographic technologist. Oxygen saturation values should be written onto the record at regular intervals and during apneic episodes. This method of display is adequate for many evaluations, but a continuous, direct recording of oxygen saturation onto the polysomnograph is clearer and more precise. Since the signal from the oximeter may be constant or only slowly varying during much of the recording, a DC amplifier is required.

Electrocardiogram

Another measurement that must be included in a complete polysomnographic recording is obtained by the ECG. The ECG may be picked up by submental or perihyoid EMG electrodes, but during periods of movement, muscle activity may obliterate the ECG tracing. The ECG may also be recorded from an impedance pneumography device superimposed on the chest movement tracing, but the exact cardiac rhythm may be obscured during periods of strenuous breathing. Consequently, if sufficient channels are available on the polygraph, a separate shoulder-to-shoulder recording of ECG is advisable.

APPROACH TO SOME COMMON SLEEP DISORDERS

Different types of polysomnographic studies have different technical requirements for evaluating some of the most common sleep disorders.

Nocturnal Seizures

According to the study of Gibberd and Bateson (1974), 6 percent of epileptic patients persistently have seizures only during sleep. Twice that many will have exclusively nocturnal seizures for the first six months after developing epilepsy. Consequently, this may be a serious diagnostic consideration in patients with deranged sleep even if daytime seizures have never occurred. Since there may be no witnesses or accurate reporting of a patient's nocturnal behavior, recording an actual seizure by polysomnography may be the only way to achieve the correct diagnosis with complete certainty.

In addition to confirming the diagnosis of nocturnal epilepsy by recording an ictal event, polysomnography or nocturnal electroencephalography may be helpful in other cases of suspected seizures by demonstrating interictal epileptiform activity (spikes or sharp waves) that may not be present during routine, daytime EEGs. The ability of sleep (Gibbs and Gibbs 1947; Niedermeyer and Rocca 1972) and sleep deprivation (Degen, 1980; Mattson, Pratt, and Calverley, 1965) to bring out epileptiform discharges is well recognized. In certain cases of complex partial seizures, however, 30 to 60 minutes of stage II sleep may be necessary to demonstrate even one convincing epileptiform paroxysm (Delgado-Escueta, 1979). For some patients, this may be difficult to achieve during the day, and a nocturnal study may be indicated.

The basic montage for staging sleep, which was described above, is generally not adequate for making the diagnosis of nocturnal epilepsy. The majority of patients with major motor convulsions during sleep will have secondarily generalized seizures (Janz, 1978) and may require an extensive array of scalp electrodes in order to localize the inciting focus. The total number of channels recorded will, of course, be limited by the size of the instrument. For sleep laboratories equipped with an 8- or 10-channel polygraph, it may be advisable simply to borrow a standard 16- or 18-channel EEG instrument to achieve more complete scalp coverage. The exact choice of montage should be dictated by the findings on the patient's routine EEG. If focal slow waves or sharp wave activity have been recorded, one should be sure that the involved area is well monitored during the study. Eye movements, respirations, and EMG are sometimes less important in questions of nocturnal seizure.

It is desirable for the patient's routine EEG to be reviewed, prior to polysomnography, but this may not always be possible. In such cases the technologist should apply a full set of scalp electrodes and survey the entire cortex before deciding on the montage to be employed for the remainder of the night. Clearly, the technician must be well trained in the use of EEG to diagnose epilepsy. This means being able to recognize characteristic abnormalities and select the recording montage that best demonstrates them. When the number of channels available for the study is limited, the choice of montage is of the greatest importance, and it may have to be varied during the course of the study for optimal results.

When no localizing features are present on the routine EEG, the minimal montage for 8-channel machines would generally include scalp-to-scalp temporal chains and the central derivation required for staging. It must be recognized that such a recording scheme does not give satisfactory coverage to the entire scalp, and the use of a polygraph with 16 channels is strongly urged whenever nocturnal epilepsy is a consideration. When 16 channels are available, 5 may be set aside for extracerebral measurements, leaving 11 to provide adequate coverage of the scalp. The noncephalic channels permit other diagnoses to be entertained even when epilepsy is primarily suspected. A single channel of combined oral and nasal air flow (see below) can rule out the possibility of sleep apnea, and electrodes from the leg muscles can exclude nocturnal myoclonus.

Some seizures of temporal lobe origin may show no definite abnormalities in the scalp EEG even during an ictal recording (Lieb, Walsh, Babb, et al, 1976). The exact number of such cases is open to question, but there is evidence that some of these patients can be diagnosed by the use of electrodes that record from the inferomesial surface of the temporal lobe (Delgado-Escueta, 1979). Because of their irritant effect, nasopharyngeal electrodes are not permissible for all-night recording. Sphenoidal electrodes, however, may be left in place for extended periods. These thin, stainless steel or silver wires are positioned just outside the foramen ovale. Placement is achieved by percutaneous insertion of a guide needle just anterior to the temporomandibular joint. This procedure is quite safe and generally free from complications; nonetheless, sphenoidal electrodes cannot be considered a routine technique in screening for epilepsy in the sleep laboratory.

Since slow paper speeds do not permit easy analysis of sharp transient or low-voltage fast activity, which is commonly seen in seizures emanating from the temporal lobes, large portions of a record may have to be run at a paper speed of 30 mm per second to clarify possible seizure activity. Video monitoring is especially important in evaluation of nocturnal seizures. Although a well-trained technologist is cognizant of the need to make careful behavioral observations, the opportunity to study a patient's movements repeatedly is afforded only by videotaping.

Nocturnal Myoclonus

In patients complaining of poor-quality nighttime sleep, nocturnal myoclonus is a diagnostic consideration. In such cases, it is desirable to quantify movements of the legs during the night. This can be accomplished most easily by attaching two standard EEG electrodes to the skin over the tibialis anterior and quadriceps muscles. The skin should be prepared in the usual manner with an abrasive agent and the electrodes filled with an electrolyte gel. An interelectrode distance of 2.5 to 5 cm along the long dimension of the muscle is adequate. Good fixation to the skin is imperative since these electrodes will be subjected to considerable movement. Application of collodion as described for the scalp should be adequate, but additional adhesive taping provides extra reinforcement. The lead wires from these electrodes should be lengthy, on the order of 3.5 m. As they extend from the patient's leg to torso, they should be fixed to the skin at several points with tape. The wires eventually pass posteriorly behind the neck and can be grouped with scalp electrodes to leave the bed in a single bundle. A standard AC amplifier will record surface EMG from the legs but the high-frequency filter should be increased to 90 Hz to avoid attenuating muscle activity.

Sleep Apnea

An adequate polysomnographic study of a patient with possible sleep apnea must include the measurement of two distinct respiratory values: ventilatory effort and resultant air exchange. The simple presence of apnea can be determined by recording cessation of air exchange at the nose and mouth. To make the clinically crucial distinction between central and obstructive apneas, however, ventilatory effort must also be monitored. If ventilatory effort persists or increases during an apneic episode, obstruction of the airway must be present.

Numerous methods have been devised for estimating ventilatory effort (Table 9.1). Only esophageal pressure transducers and the intercostal EMG truly and directly measure thoracic pressure or work by the subject. Other methods are indirect, monitoring thoracic and/or abdominal movement rather than pressure or direct muscle action. Simultaneous contraction of the diaphragm and chest wall muscles with the glottis closed may be associated with considerable ventilatory effort or pressure but very little thoracic or abdominal movement. As a result, upper airway obstruction may cause arrest of

Table 9.1.   Methods of Monitoring Ventilatory Effort

Direct	Indirect (Movement Monitors)
Intercostal EMG	Pneumatic devices
Esophageal balloon	Strain gauges
	Impedance devices
	Inductive devices
	Magnetometers

breathing movements with no recordable motion on thoracic and abdominal monitors. In such cases, both the esophageal pressure transducers and intercostal EMG would correctly demonstrate continued ventilatory effort that indirect monitors would not reveal. In practice, airway obstruction during sleep is associated not with isometric contraction of the chest wall and diaphragm but with paradoxical (i.e., opposite) movements of the chest and abdomen. These increase in amplitude with increased duration of apnea. This empirical finding allows use of thoracic and abdominal movement in routine studies to document continued ventilatory effort during obstructive apnea. When large numbers of central apneas are recorded and the patient is suspected clinically of having an obstructive apnea syndrome, it would be wise to perform another study using either an esophageal transducer or intercostal EMG. Decreased esophageal pressure or EMG activity would serve to confirm the presence of central apnea.

All of the ventilatory monitors described earlier can be used in clinical polysomnography. Except in unusual cases, the choice of one method over another is not crucially important since adequate data can be obtained by each. Nonetheless, considerations of cost, simplicity, applicability to investigational studies, and personal preference may dictate the selection of a particular system.

Narcolepsy

The diagnostic approach to patients with suspected narcolepsy differs from the approach to those with other sleep disorders. In suspected narcolepsy, the quality and quantity of daytime sleep are most important. Narcoleptic patients often show variations from normal in their nighttime sleep patterns but diagnostic abnormalities may not always be seen (Richardson, Carskadon, Flagg, et al, 1978; Kales, Kales, Bixler, et al, 1978). Consequently, the diagnosis is best made not by nocturnal polysomnography but by a convincing clinical history plus documentation of abnormal daytime sleep. A systematic method for investigating a patient's daytime sleep was developed by workers at the Stanford Sleep Disorder Clinic and Research Center

(Carskadon and Dement, 1977; Richardson et al, 1978). Their ingenious Multiple Sleep Latency Test provides an objective measure of a patient's sleepiness and the opportunity to record episodes of sleep-onset REM. The test is based on the premise that when given the opportunity to doze, a "sleepy" person will achieve sleep sooner (i.e., have a shorter sleep latency) than a non-sleepy person. By averaging the sleep latency for several daytime naps, a numerical measure of sleepiness can be given.

In practice, a patient is allowed to lie down and asked to try to fall asleep at five times during the day, namely 10 AM, 12 noon, 2 PM, 4 PM, and 6 PM. A simple recording montage suffices for following the patient's state of arousal: two EEG channels (O_1-A_2, C_3-A_2, one EMG channel (submental), and two EOG channels (ROC,-A_2, LOC'-A_2) are adequate. When sleep occurs, the time from the start of the nap is recorded as the sleep latency. Sleep is staged according to the standard criteria of Rechtschaffen and Kales (1968). Sleep onset may be either REM or non-REM (including stage I) in type. If no sleep occurs, the nap is terminated at 20 minutes, and the latency is recorded as 20 for that segment of the test. If sleep does occur, the patient is allowed to remain asleep for only 10 minutes. Thus the maximum length of any test period is 29 minutes, this in the case of a patient falling asleep after 19 minutes of wakefulness. After each segment of the test the subject is required to stay awake until the next scheduled nap. Normal values have been published for the Multiple Sleep Latency Test (Richardson et al, 1978), and a given patient's data can be compared if the test has been conducted in the standard manner. Sleep latencies for narcoleptics are consistently below control values. In addition, patients with polysymptomatic narcolepsy (the narcolepsy/cataplexy syndrome) show periods of REM sleep during the test. Mitler et al (1979) recorded two or more REM episodes in all of 40 narcoleptic patients so tested. Controls showed no REM sleep.

For several reasons, caution must be used when employing the Multiple Sleep Latency Test to diagnose narcolepsy. First, sleep apnea may coexist with narcolepsy and go unrecognized unless nocturnal polysomnography is also performed. In a series of 235 consecutive patients referred to the Stanford Sleep Disorder Clinic for excessive daytime somnolence, 10 were found to have evidence of both narcolepsy and sleep apnea (Guilleminault and Dement, 1977). Second, prior sleep deprivation of any cause will produce erroneous results on a multiple sleep latency test. Persons seeking stimulant medication can falsely lower their sleep latencies by staying awake during the night before their test. In questionable cases it may be wise to document a full night's sleep by polysomnography before this test is performed. Third, medications can confound the test. Many medications cause drowsiness as a side effect, and REM-suppressive medications may lead to excessive REM sleep in the withdrawal period (REM rebound). Reliable test results will be obtained if the patient can be maintained drug free for a week before the study.

Impotence

The clinical sleep laboratory is being called upon more and more to assist clinicians in the evaluation of men with the complaint of impotence. For years, urologists have had to rely heavily on subjective reports from the patient about his erectile function. Now, with the availability of nocturnal penile tumescence (NPT) studies, a more objective evaluation is possible.

The basic problem facing clinicians is to decide whether a patient's failure of sexual performance is psychogenic or the result of somatic disease. The presence of an erection on morning awakening has been generally regarded as sufficient evidence to exclude a somatic disorder as the cause of impotence. This criterion is flawed both because many sexually competent men do *not* experience morning erection, and because some organically impaired men may be able to have morning erections and yet not be able to achieve turgidity sufficient for intercourse. By studying penile tumescence over the course of two or three nights, a more complete and quantitative assessment of erectile function can be made.

The method relies on strain gauges that sense changes in penile circumference (Bohlen, 1981). These devices are similar in principle to those used for monitoring thoracic and abdominal movements described under the discussion of sleep apnea. Thin rubber tubes are filled with mercury or a gallium-indium alloy. Lengthening of the tube causes an increase in resistance through the strain gauge, which may be detected by a Wheatstone bridge circuit. The output of the bridge is recorded through a DC-coupled amplifier, generally on a polygraph that has very low paper speeds available.

In practice, two strain gauges are generally employed, one at the base and the other just proximal to the glans penis (Karacan, 1982). Several sizes are commercially available so that gauges may be chosen to fit snugly with the penis in the flaccid state. Prior to the study the amplifier signals are calibrated by applying the gauges to cylinders of known circumference.

In addition to penile tumescence, values for the staging of sleep are recorded; namely C_3-A_2, LOC'-A_2, ROC,-A_2, and submental EMG. Although penile tumescence may occur in the absence of REM sleep, the presence of a normally structured night's sleep strengthens the validity of an NPT study. Furthermore, the recording of a REM episode significantly earlier than expected may serve as corroborative evidence in making the diagnosis of endogenous depression.

The mere presence or absence of nocturnal erections is readily ascertainable from the recording system described. Considerably more difficult is assessment of the strength of an erection. After penile circumference has reached a maximum, further blood flow may increase turgidity significantly without causing any change in the strain gauge tracings. Therefore investigators have had to look for a more direct means of assessing penile rigidity. One method is to wake the patient during a time of apparently maximal tumescence and have him quantify the strength of this erection in comparison to the best erection he has had in the past. A more objective method requires the use of a tonometer. This device measures applied force when pressed onto the glans along the long axis of the penis. The measurement is recorded directly on the polygraph through an AC amplifier at the time of testing erectile strength. At the moment when the penile shaft buckles, the tracing will show an abrupt change. The buckling force is recorded at that point. The minimal rigidity necessary for vaginal penetration corresponds to a buckling force of about 450 gm (Karacan, 1982). One design for a tonometer has recently been published (Hahn and Leder, 1980).

If on the first night of an NPT study, a normal pattern of erection is recorded and maximal rigidity is deemed adequate for intercourse, further recordings are superfluous. When equivocal results are obtained, the possibility of a first-night effect must be entertained. Jovanovic (1969) has demonstrated the possibility of observing weaker and shorter erections on the first study night than on succeeding nights. Consequently, patients for evaluation of impotence need to have two or three nights of recording scheduled in advance.

MISCELLANEOUS TECHNIQUES

Blood Sampling

Blood sampling is not a routine procedure in clinical polysomnography, but occasionally the sleep laboratory may be called on to provide this service. In laboratories designed to study biological rhythms and disorders of the normal nychthemeral cycle, techniques have been devised for periodically sampling a subject's blood without causing arousal. Weitzman et al (1971) have described the approach used in the Sleep Disorders Center at the Albert Einstein College of Medicine. A plastic catheter is inserted into an antecubital vein prior to the start of the study. A long polyethylene tube of very narrow diameter is used to connect the catheter to a sampling port in an adjoining room. Typical dimensions of the tube are 3 m in length and 0.4 mm internal diameter. The system is kept open with a dilute solution of heparin, so prior to each sample a few milliliters of blood must be withdrawn and discarded to avoid dilution. The catheter tubing must be kept away from the subject's skin or else insulated so that the temperature difference between the flush solution and the blood sample itself will not cause arousal.

Computer Applications

At present, most sleep laboratories rely upon human scorers to analyze nocturnal polysomnograms. With the advent of relatively inexpensive digital computers, more and more of this task may be given over to machines.

Programs have been designed to analyze EEG, EOG, and EMG data, much as a human scorer does (Smith, Karacan, and Yang, 1978; Martin, Johnson, Viglione et al, 1972; Gaillard and Tissot, 1973). The computer divides the recording into time intervals of a predetermined length called epochs. The frequency characteristics of the EEG are examined for the amount of alpha, beta, and delta activity present. Special detectors also count the number of sleep spindles. The EOG channels are examined for rapid eye movements, and the level of muscle activity in the EMG channel is also taken into account.

Scoring is achieved by applying criteria similar to those of Rechtschaffen and Kales (1968). Using these criteria, agreement among human scorers is generally greater than 90 percent and often is around 95 percent. With computer programs reported in the literature, agreement between man and machine has not yet reached 85 percent. The apparent reason for this discrepancy is that human scorers intuitively make certain adjustments that are not explicitly stated in the standard rules for staging sleep. The scoring of a particular epoch is influenced by the characteristics of neighboring epochs more than the rules would seem to dictate. The variability of key waveforms with age also contributes to disagreement between human and computer staging. Smith et al (1978) have suggested that greater concordance could be achieved by changing the value settings in their scoring criteria according to the subject's age.

For the future, we may expect increased use of computers in the analysis of sleep data. Not only does automation promise to reduce the amount of human work involved in scoring polysomnograms, but it will provide quantitative information and a degree of objectivity that are presently not available.

Actigraphy

Although EEG criteria are likely to remain the definitive standard by which the architecture of sleep is judged, movement monitoring may prove to be an advantageous alternative under certain circumstances. When the only measurements of interest are the total amounts of sleep and wake time or the number of arousals, a portable movement monitor may suffice.

The technique of studying sleep by monitoring a subject's movement activity is called actigraphy. The method requires that only a single, lightweight device be strapped to the wrist or dorsum of the dominant hand. Any movement of the limb affects a piezoelectric transducer within the device, and a small electrical signal is produced. This signal can be recorded directly on a polygraph in the sleep laboratory or onto a cassette of electronic tape for studies performed in a subject's home or hospital room. The resultant tracing is subdivided into epochs of about 30 seconds and each epoch is judged to represent sleep or wakefulness depending upon the amount of movement present.

Such a system has been used successfully in estimating sleep time for both healthy subjects and patients with abnormal sleep (Mullaney, Kripke, and Messin, 1980). Using only the presence of movement to distinguish sleep from wakefulness, agreement with EEG data has been reported to be surprisingly good—greater than 90 percent of epochs are concordant. In general, however, this method has been found to overestimate total sleep time. Periods of quiet wakefulness that are readily apparent on EEG tracings are incorrectly scored as sleep when movement criteria alone are employed. The technique allows only the presence or absence of sleep to be determined. Sleep cannot be divided into REM and non-REM stages. These disadvantages are significant but in certain cases they may be outweighed by other considerations. Since this technique can be applied to at-home studies, its chief advantage is its low cost when compared to polysomnography. In addition, the devices are less cumbersome and less uncomfortable to the patient than the usual array of electrodes that are employed for monitoring sleep even when the study is performed at home. It is likely therefore that actigraphic monitors disturb sleep less than do conventional devices. It may be that more reliable and reproducible studies can be obtained through this less obtrusive method.

When an estimation of REM sleep time is also required, eye-movement monitors can be employed in conjunction with actigraphic monitors. The method of using small piezoelectric transducers to record eye movements has recently been described. This merely involves taping a single transducer to one eyelid. The output of the transducer is recorded similarly to the output of the hand-movement monitor. This system has been tested in healthy subjects, but its applicability to clinical sleep studies has yet to be determined (Kayed, Hesla, and Rosjo, 1979).

REFERENCES

Agnew H Jr, Wilse B, Williams R. The first night effect—an EEG study of sleep. Psychophysiology 1966;2:263–66.

Ashutosh K, Gilbert R, Auchinclos J, Erlebacher J, Peppi D. Impedance pneumograph and magnetometer methods for monitoring tidal volume. J Appl Physiol 1974;37:964–66.

Bohlen J. Sleep erection monitoring in the evaluation of male erectile failure. Urol Clin North Am 1981;8:119–34.

Carskadon M, Dement WC. Sleep tendency—an objective measure of sleep loss. Sleep Res 1977;6:200.

Cohn M, Watson H, Weisshaut R, Stott F, Sackner M. A transducer for non-invasive monitoring of respiration. In: Stott F. et al, eds., ISAM 1977, 2nd International Symposium on Ambulatory Monitoring. London: Academic Press, 1978:119–28.

Cooper R, Osselton J, Shaw J. EEG technology. 3rd ed. London and Boston: Butterworths, 1980;159.

Degen R. A study of the diagnostic value of waking and sleep deprivation on epileptic patients on anticonvulsant therapy. Electroencephalogr Clin Neurophysiol 1980;49:577–84.

Delgado-Escueta AV. Epileptogenic paroxysms—modern approaches and clinical correlations. Neurology (NY) 1979;29:1014–22.

Fisher J, Garza G, Flickinger R, de la Pena A. An alternate method of recording airflow during sleep. Sleep 1980;2:461–63.

Gaillard J, Tissot R. Principles of automated analysis of sleep records with a hybrid system. Comput Biomed Res 1973;6:1–13.

Gibberd F, Bateson M. Sleep epilepsy—its pattern and prognosis. Br Med J 1974;2:403–5.

Gibbs E, Gibbs F. Diagnostic and localizing value of EEG studies in sleep. Res Publ Assoc Res Nerv Ment Dis 1947;26:366–76.

Gillies A, Larkin J, Guy H. NZ Med J 1981;93:297–98.

Guilleminault WC, Dement WC. 235 cases of excessive sleepiness. J Neurol Sci 1977;31:13–27.

Hahn P, Leder R. Quantification of penile "buckling" force. Sleep 1980;3:95–97.

Hord D. Common mode rejection techniques in conjugate eye movement recording during sleep. Psychophysiology 1975;12:354–55.

Jacobson A, Kales A, Zweizig J, Kales J. Special EEG and EMG techniques for sleep research. Am J EEG Technol 1965;5:5–10.

Janz D. Epilepsy and the Sleeping-Waking Cycle. In: Vinken PJ, Bruyn GW, eds. Handbook of clinical neurology. Amsterdam: Elsevier, 1978.

Jovanovic U. Der Effect der ersten Untersuchungsnacht auf die Erektionen im Schlaf. Psychother Psychosom 1969;7:295–308.

Kales A, Kales J, Bixler E, Brennan R, Djoko M, Kerr B. Nocturnal sleep and daytime nap recordings—clinical implications. Sleep Res 1978;7:234.

Karacan I. Evaluation of NPT and impotence. In: Guilleminault C, ed., Sleeping and waking disorders—indications and techniques. Menlo Park, Calif.: Addison-Wesley, 1982.

Kayed K, Hesla P, Rosjo D. The actioculographic monitor of sleep. Sleep 1979;2:253–60.

Konno K, Mead J. Measurement of the separate volume changes of rib cage and abdomen during breathing. J Appl Physiol 1967;2:407–22.

Krumpe P, Cummiskey J. Use of laryngeal sound recordings to monitor apnea. Am Rev Respir Dis 1980;122:797–801.

Lieb J, Walsh G, Babb T, Walte R, Crandall P. A comparison of EEG seizure patterns recorded with surface and depth electrodes in patients with temporal lobe epilepsy. Epilepsia 1976;17:137–60.

Martin W, Johnson L, Viglione S, Naitoh P, Joseph R, Moses J. Pattern recognition of EEG-EOG as a technique for all-night sleep stage scoring. Electroencephalogr Clin Neurophysiol 1972;32:417–27.

Mattson R, Pratt K, Calverley J. Electroencephalograms of epileptics following sleep deprivation. Arch Neurol 1965;13:310–15.

Mendels J, Hawkins D. Sleep laboratory adaptation in normal subjects and depressed patients (first night effect). Electroencephalogr Clin Neurophysiol 1967;22:556.

Mitler M, Van Den Hoed J, Carskadon M, et al. REM sleep episodes during the multiple sleep latency test in narcoleptic patients. Electroencephalogr Clin Neurophysiol 1979;46:479–81.

Mullaney D, Kripke D, Messin S. Wrist-actigraphic estimation of sleep time. Sleep 1980;3:83–92.

Niedermeyer E, Rocca U. The diagnostic significance of sleep electroencephalograms in temporal lobe epilepsy. Eur Neurol 1972;7:119–29.

Pacela A. Impedance pneumography—a survey of instrumentation techniques. Med Biol Eng 1981;4:1–15.

Rechtschaffen A, Kales A. A manual of standardized terminology; techniques and scoring for sleep stages of human subjects. NIH Publication no. 204. Bethesda, Md.: National Institutes of Health, 1968.

Rechtschaffen A, Verdone P. Amount of dreaming—effect of incentive, adaptation to laboratory, and individual differences. Percept Motor Skills 1964;19:9–47.

Richardson G, Carskadon M, Flagg W, Van Den Hoed J, Dement WC, Mitler M. Excessive daytime sleepiness in man—multiple sleep latency measurements in narcoleptic and control subjects. Electroencephalogr Clin Neurophysiol 1978;45:621–27.

Riley T, Peterson H. Sleep studies in the subject's home. Presented at the annual scientific meeting of the American EEG Society, Chicago, June 1981.

Rosekind M, Coates T, Thorensen C. Telephone transmission of polysomnographic data from subjects' homes. J Nerv Ment Dis 1978;166:438–41.

Schmidt H, Kaelbling R. The differential laboratory adaptation of sleep parameters. Biol Psychiatry 1971;3:33–45.

Shapiro A, Cohen H. The use of mercury capillary length gauges for the measurement of the volume of thoracic and diaphragmatic components of human respiration—a theoretical analysis and practical method. Ann NY Acad Sci 1965;27:634.

Smith J, Karacan I, Yang M. Automated analysis of the human sleep EEG. Waking Sleep 1978;2:75–82.

Watson H. The technology of respiratory inductive plethysmography. In: Stott F. et al, eds., ISAM 1979, 3rd International Symposium on Ambulatory Monitoring. London: Academic Press, 1980:537–63.

Weitzman E, Fukushima D, Nogeire C, Roffusarg H, Gallagher T, Hellman L. Twenty-four-hour pattern of the episodic secretion of cortisol in normal subjects. J Clin Endocrinol 1971;33:14–22.

Wells D, Allen R, Wagman A. A single-channel system for recording eye movements. Psychophysiology 1977;14:73–74.

Wilkinson R, Mullaney D. Electroencephalogram recording of sleep in the home. Postgrad Med J 1976;52(Suppl 7):92–96.

A SLEEP GLOSSARY

Active sleep: A term used occasionally for rapid eye movement sleep, because of increased phasic movements and an appearance of activation or agitation.

Activity: An often-abused word denoting an identifiable type of waveform on EEG. Signifies groups or clusters of brain waves, and sometimes implies homogeneity. Examples: used with seizure discharges (seizure activity) or particular frequencies of waves (alpha activity).

Alpha rhythm: An independent, usually sinusoidal, type of EEG rhythm in the 8- to 13-Hz (cycles per second) frequency range. Most prominent in posterior head regions, usually disappearing when eyes are opened. Alpha rhythm is diminished in amplitude with attention or agitation, and usually attenuates with drowsiness. Dropout of alpha rhythm is one of the signs of early stage I sleep. Sometimes alpha rhythm may be seen in REM.

APSS: Association for the Psychophysiological Study of Sleep.

Artifact: A signal appearing on the graph paper not derived from the organ in study, i.e., a waveform on EEG not coming from the brain. Some would actually use the term only to refer to "nonbiological signals." Electrocardiograph impulse, eye movements of a certain type, and muscle signals, however, are all sometimes called artifact because they may be confused with brain waves or other signals in a study.

Attenuation: Diminution in voltage of a recorded signal, diminished recordability of a particular type of biological activity (for example, attenuation of an alpha rhythm with eye opening).

Background activity: A term used variably by different electroencephalographers. Usually, it refers to the basically continuous group of frequencies and activity level in the ongoing EEG, and is used to contrast with focal or episodic cerebral signals. Some authors, however, use the term to refer specifically to alpha rhythm.

Beta or beta rhythm: A frequency band of EEG rhythm more rapid than 13 Hz. Some authors restrict the term to cerebral activities with frequencies faster than 13 Hz when located only in frontal regions. Beta rhythms, as other cerebral rhythms on EEG, may or may not be synchronous or symmetrical over the two hemispheres.

Body movement: An obvious term in general parlance but scored as a specific behavior at times, especially in EEG/sleep recordings when amplitude of the EMG channel increases for more than one second or when muscle artifact voltage obliterates the EEG or EOG tracing.

Bursts: An explosive increase in activity or voltage (for example, bursts of spikes and waves). The word does not simply denote a rapid change in voltage or activity, but implies an eruption, suddenness, or dramatic quality.

Canthus: The angle or lateral margin of the eye.

Delta or delta rhythm: Term used to describe slow waves on EEG; that is, cerebral waves recorded on EEG with frequency slower than 4 Hz. Often interpreted to imply high voltage, but voltage actually is not a criterion. Delta waves may sometimes be low in voltage, depending on the circumstance of their detection on EEG. Requires very "tolerant" slow-frequency filters, in other words, long time constants in the slow-frequency filter.

Delta sleep: Often used as a synonym for stages III and IV sleep. Also called slow wave sleep. See text discussion of sleep stages.

Depth electrode or depth EEG (also called stereoencephalography): Cerebral electrical activity recorded from electrodes placed into the substance of the brain, usually in subcortical structures. The term is also used to refer to electrodes placed in sulci to reach cortical surfaces not accessible to routine scalp electrodes.

Desynchronized sleep: A synonym for REM sleep, because the EEG has a desynchronized or nonrhythmical quality. The desynchronized EEG is generally considered a sign of approaching or achieving the alert state.

Diffuse or nonfocal: When used in discussions of physiological recording or EEG, represents activities or functions that occur over large areas or may branch to large areas. Usually represents functions that occur more or less simultaneously on various scalp regions, but not necessarily in a synchronous manner.

Driving or driving response: Rhythms or functions occurring in response to a repetitive or continuous stimulus. Most often refers to flashing lights with EEG. The photic driving response is a rhythmical response to flashing lights, primarily in the occipital regions. Individual wave responses have similarities to evoked cerebral responses.

Drowsiness or drowsy stage: In some descriptions, the term drowsiness or drowsy is used to denote the state of relaxation during which alpha rhythms or alpha waves are visible. For the most part, drowsiness is considered to be a synonym for stage I sleep. It is generally characterized by the disappearance of alpha rhythm. Behaviorally, persons in stage I sleep will usually state that they felt "drowsy" but usually will deny being "asleep."

Electrical silence or electrocerebral silence: No definable electrical activity. A difficult expression, because the ambient electrical "noise" level in most laboratories or hospital buildings contains electromagnetic waveforms of sufficient voltage to cause deflections in most EEG machines. Usually the term applies to circumstances in which no recordable activity can be ascribed directly to the brain. In other words, even in conditions of unequivocal brain death, the EEG usually will record some deflections due to noncerebral physiological responses or to ambient electrical activity; this still can be considered electrocerebral silence.

Electrocorticogram (ECoG):   A recording of EEG or electrical activity derived from electrodes placed directly on the cortex of the brain.

Electroencephalogram (EEG):   A recording, usually on graph paper, of recurrent and usually alternating electrical activity generated by the brain or the brain surface. Recordings from several different surfaces on the brain are generally included, so that the EEG usually has several channels or leads. These channels represent different surfaces of the scalp and different portions of the brain underlying the scalp. It is important to recognize that electrodes placed on the scalp also record other electrical biological functions, many of which are not derived from the brain. These include electrocardiogram, eye movements, facial muscle, and movements of the tongue.

Electromyogram (EMG):   The electrical activity of muscles recorded by an oscilloscope, polygraph, or EEG machine. In sleep recordings (polysomnograms), the most commonly recorded muscles are those of the face, particularly of the mentalis muscle on the chin. Occasionally, some somatic muscles, especially the tibialis anterior in the legs, are recorded. EMG (by its disappearance) is particularly important for denoting onset of REM.

Electro-oculogram (EOG):   Recording of eye movements by their electrical signatures. There is a large dipole, often over 200 μV, between the retina (negative charge) and the cornea (positive charge) so that any movements of the eye cause movement of the dipole and can be recorded by electrodes on the face or forehead. Blinking causes a large surface-positive effect in the frontal portions of the head. EOG is especially important for gauging the onset of stage I (because of the rolling eye movements) or REM (clusters of rapid eye movements) sleep.

Fast sleep: A term, now generally abandoned, used in the past to refer to REM because of the rapid EEG frequencies during REM.

Hypnagogic: Events or circumstances occurring in the process of falling asleep. For example, hypnagogic hallucinations are those occurring in drowsiness while falling asleep.

Hypnapompic or hypnopompic: Events that occur in the process of awakening. Often used to describe seizures that occur during or immediately after awakening.

Index or phase index: The fraction or percentage of time occupied by a particular form or phase of physiological activity. Usually specified with amplitude or frequency characteristics that designate the indexed activity in a given time duration sample; e.g., REM index, representing the fraction of a brief interval during which actual rapid eye movements were occurring, or alpha index, the percentage of a given epoch during which alpha waves of a defined amplitude actually occurred.

K-Complex: EEG waveforms with a duration exceeding 0.5 second, with a primarily surface-negative polarity, usually followed by an immediate surface-positive polarity, creating a biphasic or sometimes triphasic configuration. The K-complex usually has a blunted sharp wave appearance. Distribution over the scalp is wide over frontocentral regions. Often seen in response to sudden stimulation, especially auditory, K-complexes frequently accompany hypnagogic myoclonus. Many times, but not always, sleep spindles accompany K-complexes. Should be distinguished from vertex sharp waves. Note: Some writers use the term K-complex to refer to any high-voltage sharp wave seen in conjunction with sleep spindles. This is misleading, because vertex sharp waves that usually have durations less than 300 msec (0.3 second) have a more restricted distribution on the scalp, more nearly confined to the vertex. Sleep spindles, vertex waves, and K-complexes may be seen together at different times in an individual.

Lambda wave or lambda activity: A sharp waveform in occipital regions usually with duration less than 100 msec (0.1 second) with primarily surface-positive polarity. Lambda waves are evoked not only by visual stimulation, but require some degree of eye movement.

Lambdoid waves or POST (positive occipital sharp transients):   Occipital sharp waves on EEG indistinguishable from lambda waves (see above), but occurring in sleep. Although completely normal, they may be sharp enough and high enough in voltage to be mistaken for seizure waves. They may appear quite asymmetrical and still be normal.

Latency of each sleep stage: Time from sleep onset to the appearance of each stage. Computed as the time delay from sleep onset (usually defined as first stage II) until the onset of the specific sleep stage. Occasionally, REM latency will be defined as the time from "lights out" to the beginning of REM sleep, although in most series and in this book, REM latency is the time from initial stage II to onset of REM.

Light sleep: Often used as a synonym for stage II sleep, but sometimes to denote either stage I or II.

Montage: The manner in which various physiological activities or channels are displayed on paper. The montage defines not only the number of items recorded, but the connection sequence of electrodes to respective amplifiers and the order of their display on recording paper or electromagnetic tape.

Morphology: The shape or waveform of a recorded event, when the term is used in EEG or sleep recording. For example, the morphology of a K-complex is a biphasic blunted sharpened slow wave, whereas the morphology of an alpha rhythm is a sinusoidal waveform.

Non-REM or NREM sleep: All sleep stages other than rapid eye movement sleep, i.e., stages I, II, III, and IV. Probably an unfortunate term because it encourages lumping all sleep phases into two types, REM and "other," and ignores physiological disparity among the other stages.

Paradoxical sleep: A term usually used for REM sleep in animals. This phrase is used because the animal is deeply asleep in terms of arousability and loss of postural tone, yet seems most active in terms of phasic movements or evidence of activity.

Paroxysm: A sudden event electrographically, especially when referring to EEG activity; a cluster of waveforms or EEG behavior arising abruptly from the background, standing apart by virtue of frequency, sharpness, or voltage.

Period: Time required from beginning to end of a particular epoch or cycle of behavior. The inverse of frequency when speaking of a rhythmical or recurrent activity. For example, one second is the period of a 1 Hz (cycle per second) wave.

Phase: A particular stage, form, or level of some activity. Also used to describe the time relationship of different parts of a wave or series of waves. That is, this term denotes the relative relationship of positive and negative or upward and downward deflections of a recurrent event. For example, two waves are said to be in phase when the occurrence of negative events has the same time frame, that is, they both go up or go down in synchrony.

POSTs (positive occipital sharp transients):   A synonym for lambdoid waves.

Quiet sleep: A phrase particularly used to refer to what appears to be very inactive or deep sleep in infants or animals. This usually refers to stages II and IV, or slow wave, sleep in animals or adults. Quiet sleep has two different EEG characteristics in infants, a rhythmical slow waveform and a random-frequency lower-voltage form.

Reactivity: A quality of changing frequency, voltage, or other characteristics in response to outside stimuli. Responsiveness of the EEG frequency.

REM sleep: Rapid eye movement sleep, a stage characterized by virtual loss of postural tone or tonic muscle activity but paradoxically displaying bursts of phasic or rapid, episodic movements, especially of the eyes. Also called dream sleep because the most vivid dreams occur at this time. Other synonyms include active sleep, paradoxical sleep, and fast sleep.

Rhythm: A definable form of cerebral activity, usually referring to repetitive clusters or runs of waves with more or less constant frequency and voltage.

Saw-toothed waves: Generally a description of a particular type of theta-frequency waveform. At times this term has been used for sharp waves that occur around vertex and frontal scalp regions at times when rapid eye movements occur in REM sleep. In yet other reports, such terminology is used in a nonspecific manner to describe sharp theta waves, and still on other occasions to describe occipital waveforms that have a surface-positive polarity (POSTs).

Sleep efficiency index:　Total sleep time divided by time in bed (TST/TIB). In other words, the efficiency of total sleep while in bed, or the ratio of sleep to time in bed. If in fact a subject is trying to sleep, the efficiency of sleep should be determined by the fraction of time in bed occupied by actual sleep.

Sleep period time (SPT):　The time from first falling asleep until morning awakening. Includes that time of initial sleep, any periods of waking during the night, and all subsequent sleep until final awakening. In other words, sleep period time equals time in bed minus sleep latency.

Sleep spindles (also called sigma activity in some EEG literature):　A spindle-shaped cluster of waves with a frequency between 12 and 14 Hz, a characteristic finding of stage II sleep. Scalp distribution in frontocentral regions bilaterally.

Slow wave sleep (SWS):　A stage of sleep characterized by high-voltage slow waves of delta waves on the EEG. Synonyms are stages III and IV sleep.

Sleep onset latency:　Computed differently in different laboratories. Conventionally, sleep onset latency is computed from "lights out" until the onset of stage II because spindles seen in stage II constitute visible, reliable criteria of sleep stage. Some laboratories compute sleep onset latency as the beginning of stage I or the disappearance of alpha rhythm.

Spike:　An EEG term for abrupt high-voltage waveform standing out from background activity with a needle or spike configuration. By convention, the term is usually confined to waves lasting less than 80 msec and having voltage greater than 100 µV.

Spike and wave:　An EEG configuration juxtaposing a spike and a slow wave. Strictly speaking, the term should be confined only to spike-wave complexes without an intervening plateau or gap.

Spindle sleep:　A synonym for stage II sleep, characterized by prominent sleep spindles. In addition, K-complexes and vertex waves occur in stage II.

Stage B:　A term sometimes used for stage I sleep (by this terminology, wakefulness would be stage A).

Stage C:　A synonym for stage II, or spindle, sleep.

Stage D:　A synonym for stage III sleep, delta wave sleep, with less than 50 percent of a period occupied by high-voltage delta waves.

Stage E:　A synonym for stage IV sleep, during which the EEG is fully occupied by high-voltage delta waves.

Stage sequencing:　The sequence or pattern derived in the sequential development of various sleep stages. Most individuals have a norm that is reasonably consistent from one night to another.

Stage W (wakefulness): Waking stage, with posterior 8- to 13-Hz (alpha waves) activity on the EEG and low-voltage mixed frequency activity in other scalp regions.

Stage I: A stage of electrographic sleep during which the individual may feel awake. Slow, rolling eye movements; EMG is preserved; daydreams occur.

Stage II: A stage during which responsiveness and recall are diminished but dreams may occur. Individuals often feel as though they are awake during stage II sleep. Characterized by vertex sharp waves, K-complexes, and central or bifrontal spindle waveforms in the 12- to 14-Hz range.

Stage III: A form of slow wave sleep. Used when 50 percent or less of the record is occupied by delta waves of voltage above 75 μV.

Stage IV: The slow wave sleep during which the entire EEG, or at least more than 50 percent, is occupied by delta waves of voltage equal to or greater than 75 μV.

Theta: An EEG term used to describe brain waves with frequency between 4 and 8 Hz.

Time in bed (TIB): The time from going to bed in preparation for sleep until arising from bed in the morning. Usually computed from "lights out" until a decision is made to arise from bed in the morning. This includes the latency before falling asleep and the period of wakefulness before arising in the morning. In other words, TIB is the entire time in which sleep is desired or attempted.

Time constant: A characteristic of an electronic filter that affects frequency response. Most often considered with low-frequency filters in EEG. Time constant is the mathematical product of resistance times capacitance, which is measured in units of time (most often seconds or fractions of seconds). Practically, applies to alternating-current filters.

Topography: Distribution over the surface. In describing EEG or sleep recordings, refers to the areas over the scalp from which certain waveforms or frequencies are recordable.

Total sleep time (TST): The total time of being asleep during the night. The TST equals time in bed minus sleep latency minus time awake after falling asleep minus wakefulness before arising from bed. The TST also equals sleep period time minus duration of nocturnal awakenings.

Vertex sharp waves: Sharp waves, usually briefer than 300 msec, with maximum voltage at the vertex and with a scalp projection seldom extending more than 4 cm away from the vertex; a smaller scalp distribution than K-complexes. Particularly in children, these sharp waves may be confused with epileptiform spikes.

Zeitgeber: A time clue. A sign, noise, or event in the environment notifying the organism of the relative time.

INDEX

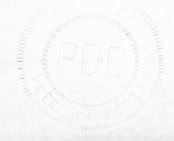